THE OFFICIAL PATIENT'S SOURCEBOOK

on

VITILIGO

JAMES N. PARKER, M.D.
AND PHILIP M. PARKER, PH.D., EDITORS

ICON Health Publications
ICON Group International, Inc.
4370 La Jolla Village Drive, 4th Floor
San Diego, CA 92122 USA

Last digit indicates print number: 10 9 8 7 6 4 5 3 2 1

Publisher, Health Care: Tiffany LaRochelle
Editor(s): James Parker, M.D., Philip Parker, Ph.D.

Publisher's note: The ideas, procedures, and suggestions contained in this book are not intended as a substitute for consultation with your physician. All matters regarding your health require medical supervision. As new medical or scientific information becomes available from academic and clinical research, recommended treatments and drug therapies may undergo changes. The authors, editors, and publisher have attempted to make the information in this book up to date and accurate in accord with accepted standards at the time of publication. The authors, editors, and publisher are not responsible for errors or omissions or for consequences from application of the book, and make no warranty, expressed or implied, in regard to the contents of this book. Any practice described in this book should be applied by the reader in accordance with professional standards of care used in regard to the unique circumstances that may apply in each situation, in close consultation with a qualified physician. The reader is advised to always check product information (package inserts) for changes and new information regarding dose and contraindications before taking any drug or pharmacological product. Caution is especially urged when using new or infrequently ordered drugs, herbal remedies, vitamins and supplements, alternative therapies, complementary therapies and medicines, and integrative medical treatments.

Cataloging-in-Publication Data

Parker, James N., 1961-
Parker, Philip M., 1960-

   The Official Patient's Sourcebook on Vitiligo: A Revised and Updated Directory for the Internet Age/James N. Parker and Philip M. Parker, editors
                p.   cm.
   Includes bibliographical references, glossary and index.
   ISBN: 0-597-83211-0
   1. Vitiligo-Popular works.   I. Title.

Disclaimer

This publication is not intended to be used for the diagnosis or treatment of a health problem or as a substitute for consultation with licensed medical professionals. It is sold with the understanding that the publisher, editors, and authors are not engaging in the rendering of medical, psychological, financial, legal, or other professional services.

References to any entity, product, service, or source of information that may be contained in this publication should not be considered an endorsement, either direct or implied, by the publisher, editors or authors. ICON Group International, Inc., the editors, or the authors are not responsible for the content of any Web pages nor publications referenced in this publication.

Copyright Notice

Dedication

To the healthcare professionals dedicating their time and efforts to the study of vitiligo.

Acknowledgements

The collective knowledge generated from academic and applied research summarized in various references has been critical in the creation of this sourcebook which is best viewed as a comprehensive compilation and collection of information prepared by various official agencies which directly or indirectly are dedicated to vitiligo. All of the *Official Patient's Sourcebooks* draw from various agencies and institutions associated with the United States Department of Health and Human Services, and in particular, the Office of the Secretary of Health and Human Services (OS), the Administration for Children and Families (ACF), the Administration on Aging (AOA), the Agency for Healthcare Research and Quality (AHRQ), the Agency for Toxic Substances and Disease Registry (ATSDR), the Centers for Disease Control and Prevention (CDC), the Food and Drug Administration (FDA), the Healthcare Financing Administration (HCFA), the Health Resources and Services Administration (HRSA), the Indian Health Service (IHS), the institutions of the National Institutes of Health (NIH), the Program Support Center (PSC), and the Substance Abuse and Mental Health Services Administration (SAMHSA). In addition to these sources, information gathered from the National Library of Medicine, the United States Patent Office, the European Union, and their related organizations has been invaluable in the creation of this sourcebook. Some of the work represented was financially supported by the Research and Development Committee at INSEAD. This support is gratefully acknowledged. Finally, special thanks are owed to Tiffany LaRochelle for her excellent editorial support.

About the Editors

James N. Parker, M.D.

Dr. James N. Parker received his Bachelor of Science degree in Psychobiology from the University of California, Riverside and his M.D. from the University of California, San Diego. In addition to authoring numerous research publications, he has lectured at various academic institutions. Dr. Parker is the medical editor for the *Official Patient's Sourcebook* series published by ICON Health Publications.

Philip M. Parker, Ph.D.

Philip M. Parker is the Eli Lilly Chair Professor of Innovation, Business and Society at INSEAD (Fontainebleau, France and Singapore). Dr. Parker has also been Professor at the University of California, San Diego and has taught courses at Harvard University, the Hong Kong University of Science and Technology, the Massachusetts Institute of Technology, Stanford University, and UCLA. Dr. Parker is the associate editor for the *Official Patient's Sourcebook* series published by ICON Health Publications.

About ICON Health Publications

In addition to vitiligo, *Official Patient's Sourcebooks* are available for the following related topics:

- The Official Patient's Sourcebook on Acne
- The Official Patient's Sourcebook on Acne Rosacea
- The Official Patient's Sourcebook on Atopic Dermatitis
- The Official Patient's Sourcebook on Behçet Syndrome
- The Official Patient's Sourcebook on Epidermolysis Bullosa
- The Official Patient's Sourcebook on Lichen Sclerosus
- The Official Patient's Sourcebook on Lyme Disease
- The Official Patient's Sourcebook on Psoriasis
- The Official Patient's Sourcebook on Raynaud's Phenomenon
- The Official Patient's Sourcebook on Scleroderma
- The Official Patient's Sourcebook on Sjogren's Syndrome

To discover more about ICON Health Publications, simply check with your preferred online booksellers, including Barnes & Noble.com and Amazon.com which currently carry all of our titles. Or, feel free to contact us directly for bulk purchases or institutional discounts:

ICON Group International, Inc.
4370 La Jolla Village Drive, Fourth Floor
San Diego, CA 92122 USA
Fax: 858-546-4341
Web site: **www.icongrouponline.com/health**

Table of Contents

INTRODUCTION

Overview

Dr. C. Everett Koop, former U.S. Surgeon General, once said, "The best prescription is knowledge."[1] The Agency for Healthcare Research and Quality (AHRQ) of the National Institutes of Health (NIH) echoes this view and recommends that every patient incorporate education into the treatment process. According to the AHRQ:

> Finding out more about your condition is a good place to start. By contacting groups that support your condition, visiting your local library, and searching on the Internet, you can find good information to help guide your treatment decisions. Some information may be hard to find — especially if you don't know where to look.[2]

As the AHRQ mentions, finding the right information is not an obvious task. Though many physicians and public officials had thought that the emergence of the Internet would do much to assist patients in obtaining reliable information, in March 2001 the National Institutes of Health issued the following warning:

> The number of Web sites offering health-related resources grows every day. Many sites provide valuable information, while others may have information that is unreliable or misleading.[3]

---

[1] Quotation from http://www.drkoop.com.

[2] The Agency for Healthcare Research and Quality (AHRQ): http://www.ahcpr.gov/consumer/diaginfo.htm.

[3] From the NIH, National Cancer Institute (NCI): **http://cancertrials.nci.nih.gov/beyond/evaluating.html.**

Since the late 1990s, physicians have seen a general increase in patient Internet usage rates. Patients frequently enter their doctor's offices with printed Web pages of home remedies in the guise of latest medical research. This scenario is so common that doctors often spend more time dispelling misleading information than guiding patients through sound therapies. *The Official Patient's Sourcebook on Vitiligo* has been created for patients who have decided to make education and research an integral part of the treatment process. The pages that follow will tell you where and how to look for information covering virtually all topics related to vitiligo, from the essentials to the most advanced areas of research.

The title of this book includes the word "official." This reflects the fact that the sourcebook draws from public, academic, government, and peer-reviewed research. Selected readings from various agencies are reproduced to give you some of the latest official information available to date on vitiligo.

Given patients' increasing sophistication in using the Internet, abundant references to reliable Internet-based resources are provided throughout this sourcebook. Where possible, guidance is provided on how to obtain free-of-charge, primary research results as well as more detailed information via the Internet. E-book and electronic versions of this sourcebook are fully interactive with each of the Internet sites mentioned (clicking on a hyperlink automatically opens your browser to the site indicated). Hard copy users of this sourcebook can type cited Web addresses directly into their browsers to obtain access to the corresponding sites. Since we are working with ICON Health Publications, hard copy *Sourcebooks* are frequently updated and printed on demand to ensure that the information provided is current.

In addition to extensive references accessible via the Internet, every chapter presents a "Vocabulary Builder." Many health guides offer glossaries of technical or uncommon terms in an appendix. In editing this sourcebook, we have decided to place a smaller glossary within each chapter that covers terms used in that chapter. Given the technical nature of some chapters, you may need to revisit many sections. Building one's vocabulary of medical terms in such a gradual manner has been shown to improve the learning process.

We must emphasize that no sourcebook on vitiligo should affirm that a specific diagnostic procedure or treatment discussed in a research study, patent, or doctoral dissertation is "correct" or your best option. This sourcebook is no exception. Each patient is unique. Deciding on appropriate options is always up to the patient in consultation with their physician and healthcare providers.

Organization

This sourcebook is organized into three parts. Part I explores basic techniques to researching vitiligo (e.g. finding guidelines on diagnosis, treatments, and prognosis), followed by a number of topics, including information on how to get in touch with organizations, associations, or other patient networks dedicated to vitiligo. It also gives you sources of information that can help you find a doctor in your local area specializing in treating vitiligo. Collectively, the material presented in Part I is a complete primer on basic research topics for patients with vitiligo.

Part II moves on to advanced research dedicated to vitiligo. Part II is intended for those willing to invest many hours of hard work and study. It is here that we direct you to the latest scientific and applied research on vitiligo. When possible, contact names, links via the Internet, and summaries are provided. It is in Part II where the vocabulary process becomes important as authors publishing advanced research frequently use highly specialized language. In general, every attempt is made to recommend "free-to-use" options.

Part III provides appendices of useful background reading for all patients with vitiligo or related disorders. The appendices are dedicated to more pragmatic issues faced by many patients with vitiligo. Accessing materials via medical libraries may be the only option for some readers, so a guide is provided for finding local medical libraries which are open to the public. Part III, therefore, focuses on advice that goes beyond the biological and scientific issues facing patients with vitiligo.

Scope

While this sourcebook covers vitiligo, your doctor, research publications, and specialists may refer to your condition using a variety of terms. Therefore, you should understand that vitiligo is often considered a synonym or a condition closely related to the following:

- Depigmentation
- Hypomelanosis
- Leukoderma

In addition to synonyms and related conditions, physicians may refer to vitiligo using certain coding systems. The International Classification of Diseases, 9th Revision, Clinical Modification (ICD-9-CM) is the most commonly used system of classification for the world's illnesses. Your physician may use this coding system as an administrative or tracking tool. The following classification is commonly used for vitiligo:[4]

- 709.0 dyschromia
- 709.1 vitiligo

For the purposes of this sourcebook, we have attempted to be as inclusive as possible, looking for official information for all of the synonyms relevant to vitiligo. You may find it useful to refer to synonyms when accessing databases or interacting with healthcare professionals and medical librarians.

Moving Forward

Since the 1980s, the world has seen a proliferation of healthcare guides covering most illnesses. Some are written by patients or their family members. These generally take a layperson's approach to understanding and coping with an illness or disorder. They can be uplifting, encouraging, and highly supportive. Other guides are authored by physicians or other healthcare providers who have a more clinical outlook. Each of these two styles of guide has its purpose and can be quite useful.

As editors, we have chosen a third route. We have chosen to expose you to as many sources of official and peer-reviewed information as practical, for the purpose of educating you about basic and advanced knowledge as recognized by medical science today. You can think of this sourcebook as your personal Internet age reference librarian.

Why "Internet age"? All too often, patients diagnosed with vitiligo will log on to the Internet, type words into a search engine, and receive several Web site listings which are mostly irrelevant or redundant. These patients are left to wonder where the relevant information is, and how to obtain it. Since only the smallest fraction of information dealing with vitiligo is even indexed in

---

[4] This list is based on the official version of the World Health Organization's 9th Revision, International Classification of Diseases (ICD-9). According to the National Technical Information Service, "ICD-9CM extensions, interpretations, modifications, addenda, or errata other than those approved by the U.S. Public Health Service and the Health Care Financing Administration are not to be considered official and should not be utilized. Continuous maintenance of the ICD-9-CM is the responsibility of the federal government."

search engines, a non-systematic approach often leads to frustration and disappointment. With this sourcebook, we hope to direct you to the information you need that you would not likely find using popular Web directories. Beyond Web listings, in many cases we will reproduce brief summaries or abstracts of available reference materials. These abstracts often contain distilled information on topics of discussion.

While we focus on the more scientific aspects of vitiligo, there is, of course, the emotional side to consider. Later in the sourcebook, we provide a chapter dedicated to helping you find peer groups and associations that can provide additional support beyond research produced by medical science. We hope that the choices we have made give you the most options available in moving forward. In this way, we wish you the best in your efforts to incorporate this educational approach into your treatment plan.

The Editors

PART I: THE ESSENTIALS

ABOUT PART I

Part I has been edited to give you access to what we feel are "the essentials" on vitiligo. The essentials of a disease typically include the definition or description of the disease, a discussion of who it affects, the signs or symptoms associated with the disease, tests or diagnostic procedures that might be specific to the disease, and treatments for the disease. Your doctor or healthcare provider may have already explained the essentials of vitiligo to you or even given you a pamphlet or brochure describing vitiligo. Now you are searching for more in-depth information. As editors, we have decided, nevertheless, to include a discussion on where to find essential information that can complement what your doctor has already told you. In this section we recommend a process, not a particular Web site or reference book. The process ensures that, as you search the Web, you gain background information in such a way as to maximize your understanding.

CHAPTER 1. THE ESSENTIALS ON VITILIGO: GUIDELINES

Overview

Official agencies, as well as federally-funded institutions supported by national grants, frequently publish a variety of guidelines on vitiligo. These are typically called "Fact Sheets" or "Guidelines." They can take the form of a brochure, information kit, pamphlet, or flyer. Often they are only a few pages in length. The great advantage of guidelines over other sources is that they are often written with the patient in mind. Since new guidelines on vitiligo can appear at any moment and be published by a number of sources, the best approach to finding guidelines is to systematically scan the Internet-based services that post them.

The National Institutes of Health (NIH)[5]

The National Institutes of Health (NIH) is the first place to search for relatively current patient guidelines and fact sheets on vitiligo. Originally founded in 1887, the NIH is one of the world's foremost medical research centers and the federal focal point for medical research in the United States. At any given time, the NIH supports some 35,000 research grants at universities, medical schools, and other research and training institutions, both nationally and internationally. The rosters of those who have conducted research or who have received NIH support over the years include the world's most illustrious scientists and physicians. Among them are 97 scientists who have won the Nobel Prize for achievement in medicine.

---

[5] Adapted from the NIH: **http://www.nih.gov/about/NIHoverview.html**.

There is no guarantee that any one Institute will have a guideline on a specific disease, though the National Institutes of Health collectively publish over 600 guidelines for both common and rare diseases. The best way to access NIH guidelines is via the Internet. Although the NIH is organized into many different Institutes and Offices, the following is a list of key Web sites where you are most likely to find NIH clinical guidelines and publications dealing with vitiligo and associated conditions:

- Office of the Director (OD); guidelines consolidated across agencies available at **http://www.nih.gov/health/consumer/conkey.htm**

- National Library of Medicine (NLM); extensive encyclopedia (A.D.A.M., Inc.) with guidelines available at **http://www.nlm.nih.gov/medlineplus/healthtopics.html**

- National Institute of Arthritis and Musculoskeletal and Skin Diseases (NIAMS); fact sheets and guidelines at **http://www.nih.gov/niams/healthinfo/**

Among those listed above, the National Institute of Arthritis and Musculoskeletal and Skin Diseases (NIAMS) is especially noteworthy. The mission of NIAMS, a part of the National Institutes of Health (NIH), is to support research into the causes, treatment, and prevention of arthritis and musculoskeletal and skin diseases, the training of basic and clinical scientists to carry out this research, and the dissemination of information on research progress in these diseases. The National Institute of Arthritis and Musculoskeletal and Skin Diseases Information Clearinghouse is a public service sponsored by the NIAMS that provides health information and information sources. The NIAMS provides the following guideline concerning vitiligo.[6]

What Is Vitiligo?[7]

Vitiligo (vit-ill-EYE-go) is a pigmentation disorder in which melanocytes (the cells that make pigment) in the skin, the mucous membranes (tissues that line the inside of the mouth and nose and genital and rectal areas), and the retina (inner layer of the eyeball) are destroyed. As a result, white patches of skin appear on different parts of the body. The hair that grows in areas affected by vitiligo usually turns white.

---

[6] This and other passages are adapted from the NIH and NIAMS (**http://www.niams.nih.gov/hi/index.htm**). "Adapted" signifies that the text is reproduced with attribution, with some or no editorial adjustments.

[7] Adapted from the National Institute of Arthritis and Musculoskeletal and Skin Diseases (NIAMS): **http://www.niams.nih.gov/hi/topics/vitiligo/vitiligo.htm** .

The cause of vitiligo is not known, but doctors and researchers have several different theories. One theory is that people develop antibodies that destroy the melanocytes in their own bodies. Another theory is that melanocytes destroy themselves. Finally, some people have reported that a single event such as sunburn or emotional distress triggered vitiligo; however, these events have not been scientifically proven to cause vitiligo.

Who Is Affected by Vitiligo?

About 1 to 2 percent of the world's population, or 40 to 50 million people, have vitiligo. In the United States, 2 to 5 million people have the disorder. Ninety-five percent of people who have vitiligo develop it before their 40th birthday. The disorder affects all races and both sexes equally.

Vitiligo seems to be more common in people with certain autoimmune diseases (diseases in which a person's immune system reacts against the body's own organs or tissues). These autoimmune diseases include hyperthyroidism (an overactive thyroid gland), adrenocortical insufficiency (the adrenal gland does not produce enough of the hormone called corticosteroid), alopecia areata (patches of baldness), and pernicious anemia (a low level of red blood cells caused by failure of the body to absorb vitamin B-12). Scientists do not know the reason for the association between vitiligo and these autoimmune diseases. However, most people with vitiligo have no other autoimmune disease.

Vitiligo may also be hereditary, that is, it can run in families. Children whose parents have the disorder are more likely to develop vitiligo. However, most children will not get vitiligo even if a parent has it, and most people with vitiligo do not have a family history of the disorder.

Key Words

- Antibodies--protective proteins produced by the body's immune system to fight infectious agents (such as bacteria or viruses) or other "foreign" substances. Occasionally, antibodies develop that can attack a part of the body and cause an "autoimmune" disease. These antibodies are called autoantibodies.

- Pigment--a coloring matter in the cells and tissues of the body.

- Pigmentation--coloring of the skin, hair, mucous membranes, and retina of the eye.

- Depigmentation--loss of color in the skin, hair, mucous membranes, or retina of the eye.
- Melanin--a yellow, brown, or black pigment that determines skin color. Melanin also acts as a sunscreen and protects the skin from ultraviolet light.
- Melanocytes--special skin cells that produce melanin.
- Ultraviolet light A (UVA)--one type of radiation that is part of sunlight and reaches the earth's surface. Exposure to UVA can cause the skin to tan. Ultraviolet light is also used in a treatment called phototherapy for certain skin conditions, including vitiligo.

What Are the Symptoms of Vitiligo?

People who develop vitiligo usually first notice white patches (depigmentation) on their skin. These patches are more common in sun-exposed areas, including the hands, feet, arms, face, and lips. Other common areas for white patches to appear are the armpits and groin and around the mouth, eyes, nostrils, navel, and genitals.

Vitiligo generally appears in one of three patterns. In one pattern (focal pattern), the depigmentation is limited to one or only a few areas. Some people develop depigmented patches on only one side of their bodies (segmental pattern). But for most people who have vitiligo, depigmentation occurs on different parts of the body (generalized pattern). In addition to white patches on the skin, people with vitiligo may have premature graying of the scalp hair, eyelashes, eyebrows, and beard. People with dark skin may notice a loss of color inside their mouths.

Will the Depigmented Patches Spread?

There is no way to predict if vitiligo will spread. For some people, the depigmented patches do not spread. The disorder is usually progressive, however, and over time the white patches will spread to other areas of the body. For some people, vitiligo spreads slowly, over many years. For other people, spreading occurs rapidly. Some people have reported additional depigmentation following periods of physical or emotional stress.

How Is Vitiligo Diagnosed?

If a doctor suspects that a person has vitiligo, he or she usually begins by asking the person about his or her medical history. Important factors in a person's medical history are a family history of vitiligo; a rash, sunburn, or other skin trauma at the site of vitiligo 2 to 3 months before depigmentation started; stress or physical illness; and premature (before age 35) graying of the hair. In addition, the doctor will need to know whether the patient or anyone in the patient's family has had any autoimmune diseases and whether the patient is very sensitive to the sun. The doctor will then examine the patient to rule out other medical problems. The doctor may take a small sample (biopsy) of the affected skin. He or she may also take a blood sample to check the blood-cell count and thyroid function. For some patients, the doctor may recommend an eye examination to check for uveitis (inflammation of part of the eye). A blood test to look for the presence of antinuclear antibodies (a type of autoantibody) may also be done. This test helps determine if the patient has another autoimmune disease.

How Can People Cope with the Emotional and Psychological Aspects?

The change in appearance caused by vitiligo can affect a person's emotional and psychological well-being and may create difficulty in getting or keeping a job. People with this disorder can experience emotional stress, particularly if vitiligo develops on visible areas of the body, such as the face, hands, arms, feet, or on the genitals. Adolescents, who are often particularly concerned about their appearance, can be devastated by widespread vitiligo. Some people who have vitiligo feel embarrassed, ashamed, depressed, or worried about how others will react.

Several strategies can help a person cope with vitiligo. First, it is important to find a doctor who is knowledgeable about vitiligo and takes the disorder seriously. The doctor should also be a good listener and be able to provide emotional support. Patients need to let their doctors know if they are feeling depressed because doctors and other mental health professionals can help people deal with depression. Patients should also learn as much as possible about the disorder and treatment choices so that they can participate in making important decisions about medical care.

Talking with other people who have vitiligo may also help a person cope. The National Vitiligo Foundation can provide information about vitiligo and refer people to local chapters that have support groups of patients, families, and physicians. Family and friends are another source of support.

Some people with vitiligo have found that cosmetics that cover the white patches improve their appearance and help them feel better about themselves. A person may need to experiment with several brands of concealing cosmetics before finding the product that works best.

What Treatment Options Are Available?

The goal of treating vitiligo is to restore the function of the skin and to improve the patient's appearance. Therapy for vitiligo takes a long time--it usually must be continued for 6 to 18 months. The choice of therapy depends on the number of white patches and how widespread they are and on the patient's preference for treatment. Each patient responds differently to therapy, and a particular treatment may not work for everyone. Current treatment options for vitiligo include medical, surgical, and adjunctive therapies (therapies that can be used along with surgical or medical treatments).

Treatment Options for Vitiligo

Medical therapies:
- Topical steroid therapy
- Topical psoralen photochemotherapy
- Oral psoralen photochemotherapy
- Depigmentation

Surgical therapies:
- Skin grafts from a person's own tissues (autologous)
- Skin grafts using blisters
- Micropigmentation (tattooing)
- Autologous melanocyte transplants

Adjunctive therapies:
- Sunscreens

- Cosmetics
- Counseling and support

Medical Therapies

Topical Steroid Therapy

Steroids may be helpful in repigmenting the skin (returning the color to white patches), particularly if started early in the disease. Corticosteroids are a group of drugs similar to the hormones produced by the adrenal glands (such as cortisone). Doctors often prescribe a mild topical corticosteroid cream for children under 10 years old and a stronger one for adults. Patients must apply the cream to the white patches on their skin for at least 3 months before seeing any results. It is the simplest and safest treatment but not as effective as psoralen photochemotherapy (see below). The doctor will closely monitor the patient for side effects such as skin shrinkage and skin striae (streaks or lines on the skin).

Psoralen Photochemotherapy

Psoralen photochemotherapy (psoralen and ultraviolet A therapy, or PUVA) is probably the most beneficial treatment for vitiligo available in the United States. The goal of PUVA therapy is to repigment the white patches. However, it is time-consuming and care must be taken to avoid side effects, which can sometimes be severe. Psoralens are drugs that contain chemicals that react with ultraviolet light to cause darkening of the skin. The treatment involves taking psoralen by mouth (orally) or applying it to the skin (topically). This is followed by carefully timed exposure to ultraviolet A (UVA) light from a special lamp or to sunlight. Patients usually receive treatments in their doctors' offices so they can be carefully watched for any side effects. Patients must minimize exposure to sunlight at other times.

Topical Psoralen Photochemotherapy

Topical psoralen photochemotherapy often is used for people with a small number of depigmented patches (affecting less than 20 percent of the body). It is also used for children 2 years old and older who have localized patches of vitiligo. Treatments are done in a doctor's office under artificial UVA light once or twice a week. The doctor or nurse applies a thin coat of psoralen to the patient's depigmented patches about 30 minutes before UVA light exposure. The patient is then exposed to an amount of UVA light that turns the affected area pink. The doctor usually increases the dose of UVA light slowly over many weeks. Eventually, the pink areas fade and a more normal skin color appears. After each treatment, the patient washes his or her skin with soap and water and applies a sunscreen before leaving the doctor's office.

There are two major potential side effects of topical PUVA therapy: (1) severe sunburn and blistering and (2) too much repigmentation or darkening of the treated patches or the normal skin surrounding the vitiligo (hyperpigmentation). Patients can minimize their chances of sunburn if they avoid exposure to direct sunlight after each treatment. Hyperpigmentation is usually a temporary problem and eventually disappears when treatment is stopped.

Oral Psoralen Photochemotherapy

Oral PUVA therapy is used for people with more extensive vitiligo (affecting greater than 20 percent of the body) or for people who do not respond to topical PUVA therapy. Oral psoralen is not recommended for children under 10 years of age because of an increased risk of damage to the eyes, such as cataracts. For oral PUVA therapy, the patient takes a prescribed dose of psoralen by mouth about 2 hours before exposure to artificial UVA light or sunlight. The doctor adjusts the dose of light until the skin areas being treated become pink. Treatments are usually given two or three times a week, but never 2 days in a row.

For patients who cannot go to a PUVA facility, the doctor may prescribe psoralen to be used with natural sunlight exposure. The doctor will give the patient careful instructions on carrying out treatment at home and monitor the patient during scheduled checkups.

Known side effects of oral psoralen include sunburn, nausea and vomiting, itching, abnormal hair growth, and hyperpigmentation. Oral psoralen photochemotherapy may increase the risk of skin cancer. To avoid sunburn and reduce the risk of skin cancer, patients undergoing oral PUVA therapy should apply sunscreen and avoid direct sunlight for 24 to 48 hours after each treatment. Patients should also wear protective UVA sunglasses for 18 to 24 hours after each treatment to avoid eye damage, particularly cataracts.

Depigmentation

Depigmentation involves fading the rest of the skin on the body to match the already white areas. For people who have vitiligo on more than 50 percent of their bodies, depigmentation may be the best treatment option. Patients apply the drug monobenzylether of hydroquinone (monobenzone or Benoquin[8]) twice a day to pigmented areas until they match the already depigmented areas. Patients must avoid direct skin-to-skin contact with other people for at least 2 hours after applying the drug.

The major side effect of depigmentation therapy is inflammation (redness and swelling) of the skin. Patients may experience itching, dry skin, or abnormal darkening of the membrane that covers the white of the eye. Depigmentation is permanent and cannot be reversed. In addition, a person who undergoes depigmentation will always be abnormally sensitive to sunlight.

Surgical Therapies

All surgical therapies must be viewed as experimental because their effectiveness and side effects remain to be fully defined.

Autologous Skin Grafts

In an autologous (use of a person's own tissues) skin graft, the doctor removes skin from one area of a patient's body and attaches it to another area. This type of skin grafting is sometimes used for patients with small patches of vitiligo. The doctor removes sections of the normal, pigmented skin (donor sites) and places them on the depigmented areas (recipient sites). There are several possible complications of autologous skin grafting. Infections may occur at the donor or recipient sites. The recipient and donor sites may develop scarring, a cobblestone appearance, or a spotty pigmentation, or may fail to repigment at all. Treatment with grafting takes time and is costly, and most people find it neither acceptable nor affordable.

---

[8] Brand names are provided as examples only, and their inclusion does not mean that these products are endorsed by the National Institutes of Health or any other Government agency. Also, if a particular brand name is not mentioned, this does not mean or imply that the product is unsatisfactory.

Skin Grafts Using Blisters

In this procedure, the doctor creates blisters on the patient's pigmented skin by using heat, suction, or freezing cold. The tops of the blisters are then cut out and transplanted to a depigmented skin area. The risks of blister grafting include the development of a cobblestone appearance, scarring, and lack of repigmentation. However, there is less risk of scarring with this procedure than with other types of grafting.

Micropigmentation (Tattooing)

Tattooing implants pigment into the skin with a special surgical instrument. This procedure works best for the lip area, particularly in people with dark skin; however, it is difficult for the doctor to match perfectly the color of the skin of the surrounding area. Tattooing tends to fade over time. In addition, tattooing of the lips may lead to episodes of blister outbreaks caused by the herpes simplex virus.

Autologous Melanocyte Transplants

In this procedure, the doctor takes a sample of the patient's normal pigmented skin and places it in a laboratory dish containing a special cell culture solution to grow melanocytes. When the melanocytes in the culture solution have multiplied, the doctor transplants them to the patient's depigmented skin patches. This procedure is currently experimental and is impractical for the routine care of people with vitiligo.

Additional Therapies

Sunscreens

People who have vitiligo, particularly those with fair skin, should use a sunscreen that provides protection from both the UVA and UVB forms of ultraviolet light. Sunscreen helps protect the skin from sunburn and long-term damage. Sunscreen also minimizes tanning, which makes the contrast between normal and depigmented skin less noticeable.

Cosmetics

Some patients with vitiligo cover depigmented patches with stains, makeup, or self-tanning lotions. These cosmetic products can be particularly effective for people whose vitiligo is limited to exposed areas of the body. Dermablend, Lydia O'Leary, Clinique, Fashion Flair, Vitadye, and Chromelin offer makeup or dyes that patients may find helpful for covering up depigmented patches.

Counseling and Support Groups

Many people with vitiligo find it helpful to get counseling from a mental health professional. People often find they can talk to their counselor about issues that are difficult to discuss with anyone else. A mental health counselor can also offer patients support and help in coping with vitiligo. In addition, it may be helpful to attend a vitiligo support group.

What Research Is Being Done on Vitiligo?

For more than a decade, research on how melanocytes play a role in vitiligo has greatly increased. This includes research on autologous melanocyte transplants. At the University of Colorado, NIAMS supports a large collaborative project involving families with vitiligo in the United States and the United Kingdom. To date, over 2,400 patients are involved. It is hoped that genetic analysis of these families will uncover the location--and possibly the specific gene or genes--conferring susceptibility to the disease. Doctors and researchers continue to look for the causes of and new treatments for vitiligo.

Where Can I Get More Information about Vitiligo?

For more information, contact:

American Academy of Dermatology
930 North Meacham Road
Schaumburg, IL 60173
Phone: 847-330-0230 or
888-462-DERM (3376) (free of charge)
Fax: 847-330-0050
www.aad.org
The academy is the national organization for dermatology. It is dedicated to achieving the highest quality of dermatologic care for everyone. The academy produces patient information on vitiligo. It can also provide referrals to dermatologists.

National Vitiligo Foundation
611 South Fleishel Avenue
Tyler, TX 75701
Phone: 903-531-0074
Fax: 903-525-1234
E-mail: vitiligo@trimofran.org
www.pegasus.uthct.edu/Vitiligo/index.html
The foundation strives to locate, inform, and counsel vitiligo patients and their families; to increase public awareness and concern for the vitiligo patient; to broaden the concern for the patient within the medical community; and to encourage, promote, and fund increased scientific and clinical research on the cause, treatment, and ultimate cure.

More Guideline Sources

The guideline above on vitiligo is only one example of the kind of material that you can find online and free of charge. The remainder of this chapter will direct you to other sources which either publish or can help you find additional guidelines on topics related to vitiligo. Many of the guidelines listed below address topics that may be of particular relevance to your specific situation or of special interest to only some patients with vitiligo. Due to space limitations these sources are listed in a concise manner. Do not hesitate to consult the following sources by either using the Internet hyperlink provided, or, in cases where the contact information is provided, contacting the publisher or author directly.

Topic Pages: MEDLINEplus

For patients wishing to go beyond guidelines published by specific Institutes of the NIH, the National Library of Medicine has created a vast and patient-oriented healthcare information portal called MEDLINEplus. Within this Internet-based system are "health topic pages." You can think of a health topic page as a guide to patient guides. To access this system, log on to **http://www.nlm.nih.gov/medlineplus/healthtopics.html.** From there you can either search using the alphabetical index or browse by broad topic areas.

If you do not find topics of interest when browsing health topic pages, then you can choose to use the advanced search utility of MEDLINEplus at **http://www.nlm.nih.gov/medlineplus/advancedsearch.html.** This utility is similar to the NIH Search Utility, with the exception that it only includes material linked within the MEDLINEplus system (mostly patient-oriented information). It also has the disadvantage of generating unstructured results. We recommend, therefore, that you use this method only if you have a very targeted search.

The Combined Health Information Database (CHID)

CHID Online is a reference tool that maintains a database directory of thousands of journal articles and patient education guidelines on vitiligo and related conditions. One of the advantages of CHID over other sources is that it offers summaries that describe the guidelines available, including contact information and pricing. CHID's general Web site is **http://chid.nih.gov/.** To search this database, go to **http://chid.nih.gov/detail/detail.html.** In particular, you can use the advanced search options to look up pamphlets, reports, brochures, and information kits. The following was recently posted in this archive:

- **Guidelines for the Treatment of Patients with Vitiligo**

  Source: Tyler, TX: National Vitiligo Foundation, Inc. [6 p.].

  Contact: Available from National Vitiligo Foundation, Inc. P.O. Box 6337, Tyler, TX 75711. (903) 534-2925; FAX (903) 534-8075. PRICE: Free.

  Summary: This information packet for physicians presents guidelines from five physicians for vitiligo management and patient care. Topics include general treatment guidelines and procedures, different treatment approaches, and topical PUVA therapy procedures. Indications and contraindications for therapies and supportive care also are included in the discussions.

- **Questions and Answers About Vitiligo**

Source: Bethesda, MD: National Institute of Arthritis and Musculoskeletal and Skin Diseases (NIAMS) Information Clearinghouse. 2001. 24 p.

Contact: Available from National Institute of Arthritis and Musculoskeletal and Skin Diseases (NIAMS) Information Clearinghouse. 1 AMS Circle, Bethesda, MD 20892-3675. (877) 226-4267 or (301) 495-4484. Fax (301) 718-6366. TTY (301) 565-2966. E-mail: NIAMSInfo@mail.nih.gov. Website: www.niams.nih.gov. PRICE: 1 to 25 copies free. Order Number: AR-05QA (booklet), or AR-05L QA (large print).

Summary: This fact sheet for people with vitiligo uses a question and answer format to provide information. It describes the symptoms of this pigmentation disorder, whom it can affect, how it progresses, how a doctor makes a diagnosis, and the available options for treatment. The fact sheet emphasizes the importance of good medical, family, and other support in helping people cope with the disorder. It also describes current research on the causes and treatments for the disorder. The fact sheet then refers the reader to a list of voluntary and professional health organizations for additional information about vitiligo. A large print version of this fact sheet is also available.

- **Handbook for Schools [on] Vitiligo**

Source: Tyler, TX: National Vitiligo Foundation. 200x. 8 p.

Contact: Available from National Vitiligo Foundation. 611 South Fleishel Avenue, Tyler, TX 75701. (903) 531-0074. Fax (903) 525-1234. E-mail: vitiligo@trimofran.org. Website: www.vitiligofoundation.org. PRICE: Single copy free.

Summary: This pamphlet provides teachers with information on vitiligo. This skin disorder is characterized by the loss of skin pigment on various parts of the body. Although the cause is unknown, there is a family history of the disorder in more than half of the cases. The disorder is not serious or life threatening, but it can have an impact on social and psychological well being. Dermatologists can treat vitiligo by a combination of medication and sunlight. The pamphlet discusses the impact of vitiligo on the child of elementary school age, the early adolescent, and the adolescent. In addition, the pamphlet presents some school experiences of pupils who have vitiligo and suggests ways in which teachers can help.

- **Vitiligo**

    Source: Schaumburg, IL: American Academy of Dermatology. 1994. 4 p.

    Contact: Available from American Academy of Dermatology. P.O. Box 681069, Schaumburg, IL 60168-1069. (888) 462-3376 or (847) 330-0230. http://www.aad.org/index.html. PRICE: Single copy free; bulk prices available.

    Summary: This brochure for people with vitiligo uses a question and answer format to provide information. Vitiligo is described as a skin condition that affects 1 or 2 of every 100 people, and causes white patches to appear on the skin as a result of loss of pigment. Although the exact cause of vitiligo is unknown, the brochure outlines several theories. It also explains how the course and severity of pigment loss differ among people with the condition, and the several options for treating vitiligo. These include avoiding tanning of normal skin in fair-skinned people and disguising vitiligo with make-up, self-tanning compound, or dyes. Alternative modes of treatment are listed; sunscreen and cover-up methods are the best treatments for children with vitiligo. At the present time, no cure exists for this condition; however, research is ongoing. 2 photographs.

- **Black Skin**

    Source: Schaumburg, IL: American Academy of Dermatology. 1994. 8 p.

    Contact: Available from American Academy of Dermatology. P.O. Box 681069, Schaumburg, IL 60168-1069. (888) 462-3376 or (847) 330-0230. http://www.aad.org/index.html. PRICE: Single copy free; bulk prices available.

    Summary: This brochure for African Americans provides information on skin, hair, and nail conditions that more commonly affect this ethnic group. It explains that African Americans may experience dry skin, variations in skin color, vitiligo, pityriasis alba, dermatosis papulosa nigra, keloids, and folliculitis keloidalis. Problems with hair loss or breaking may occur as a result of certain techniques and preparations used to treat African American hair. Other hair-related conditions include tinea capitis and ingrown hairs of the beard. The brochure highlights the features of and treatments for these conditions. It also notes that African Americans should be aware that increased darkening around the base of the nail could be a sign of malignant melanoma. 7 photographs.

- **Vitiligo: A Manual for Physicians**

  Source: Tyler, TX: National Vitiligo Foundation, Inc. [8 p.].

  Contact: Available from National Vitiligo Foundation, Inc. P.O. Box 6337, Tyler, TX 75711. (903) 534-2925; FAX (903) 534-8075. PRICE: Free.

  Summary: This brochure for physicians presents general information about vitiligo, including its causes, symptoms, onset, diagnosis, and treatment. The psychological aspects of the disease, the social implications caused by skin characteristics of vitiligo, and the importance of a positive physician-patient relationship in managing the effects of the disease are discussed. Resources to contact for additional information are listed. 7 references.

- **Vitiligo: A Handbook for Schools**

  Source: Tyler, TX: National Vitiligo Foundation, Inc. [8 p.].

  Contact: Available from National Vitiligo Foundation, Inc. P.O. Box 6337, Tyler, TX 75711. (903) 534-2925; FAX (903) 534-8075. PRICE: Free.

  Summary: This brochure for school personnel presents general information about vitiligo, including its causes, symptoms, onset, and treatment. The psychosocial impact of vitiligo on elementary, middle, and high school students is discussed, as well as experiences of students in various school settings. Ways in which teachers can help students with vitiligo and their families cope with the social consequences of the disease are listed. The brochure also lists resources teachers can contact for additional information about vitiligo.

- **Vitiligo: A Handbook for Patients**

  Source: Tyler, TX: National Vitiligo Foundation, Inc. [12 p.].

  Contact: Available from National Vitiligo Foundation, Inc. P.O. Box 6337, Tyler, TX 75711. (903) 534-2925; FAX (903) 534-8075. PRICE: Free.

  Summary: This brochure presents general information about vitiligo including causes, disease progression, signs and symptoms, treatment, genetic factors, and psychosocial implications of the disease. Topics such as self care and patient support, locating additional resources and information about vitiligo, and helping adolescents and children cope with the social implications of the disease are also discussed.

- **Handbook for Patients: Vitiligo**

  Source: Tyler, TX: National Vitiligo Foundation. 199x. 16 p.

Contact: National Vitiligo Foundation. 611 South Fleishel Avenue, Tyler, TX 75701. (903) 531-0074. Fax (903) 525-1234. E-mail: vitiligo@trimofran.org. Website: www.vitiligofoundation.org. PRICE: Single copy free; donation or membership requested.

Summary: This pamphlet uses a question and answer format to provide people who have vitiligo with information on this noncontagious, noncancerous disease in which the skin loses pigment as a result of the destruction of pigment cells. Skin in body folds, around body openings, and on the hands and face are the most common sites of pigment loss. Although vitiligo is common in the general population, its incidence is higher in people with thyroid conditions and some other metabolic diseases. The cause of vitiligo is unknown, but it may have a hereditary component. Vitiligo may spread to other areas of the body; however, there is no way of predicting whether or where it will spread. The symptoms of vitiligo can be treated with a combination of a drug called psoralen and regulated doses of sunlight. Total depigmentation may be attempted in severe cases of vitiligo to give the patient an even color. Cosmetic coverups may also be effective in minimizing the visibility of vitiligo. The disease should not interfere with interpersonal relations, even intimate ones, if people who have vitiligo have a healthy self image and seek relationships with people who value more than superficial appearance. The pamphlet offers advice to junior high school students who have vitiligo and the parents of children who have the disease. In addition, sources of information about the disease are identified.

- **About Vitiligo**

Source: Tyler, TX: National Vitiligo Foundation. 199x. 8 p.

Contact: National Vitiligo Foundation. 611 South Fleishel Avenue, Tyler, TX 75701. (903) 531-0074. Fax (903) 525-1234. E-mail: vitiligo@trimofran.org. Website: www.vitiligofoundation.org. PRICE: Single copy free; donation or membership requested.

Summary: This pamphlet uses a question and answer format to provide information to people who have vitiligo. In this disease, the skin loses pigment as a result of the destruction of pigment cells. Common sites of pigment loss include skin in body folds; skin around body openings; and skin on the hands, face, and other exposed areas. People who have vitiligo face a greater risk of having hyperthyroidism, hypothyroidism, pernicious anemia, Addison's disease, alopecia areata, and uveitis. The cause of vitiligo is unknown, but it may have hereditary, immunologic, and neurogenic components. Vitiligo may begin with a rapid loss of pigment which is followed by a lengthy period when the skin color does not change. However, there is no way of predicting whether or where vitiligo will spread. The basic methods of treating vitiligo are restoring the normal pigment or destroying the remaining pigment. In repigmentation therapy, the patient is given psoralen and then exposed to ultraviolet light. Total depigmentation may be attempted in severe cases of vitiligo to give the patient an even color. Cosmetic coverups may also be effective in minimizing the visibility of vitiligo. The pamphlet outlines the requirements for repigmentation therapy and highlights the activities of the National Vitiligo Foundation.

The National Guideline Clearinghouse™

The National Guideline Clearinghouse™ offers hundreds of evidence-based clinical practice guidelines published in the United States and other countries. You can search their site located at **http://www.guideline.gov/** by using the keyword "vitiligo" or synonyms.

Healthfinder™

Healthfinder™ is an additional source sponsored by the U.S. Department of Health and Human Services which offers links to hundreds of other sites that contain healthcare information. This Web site is located at **http://www.healthfinder.gov**. Again, keyword searches can be used to find guidelines. The following was recently found in this database:

- **Questions and Answers About Vitiligo**

  Summary: An online consumer health information document that provides basic information on this pigmentation disorder.

  Source: National Institute of Arthritis and Musculoskeletal and Skin Diseases, National Institutes of Health

  http://www.healthfinder.gov/scripts/recordpass.asp?RecordType=0&RecordID=2252

- **Vitiligo**

  Summary: Consumer health information fact sheet about this autoimmune skin condition that is characterized by white patches resulting from loss of pigment.

  Source: American Academy of Dermatology

  http://www.healthfinder.gov/scripts/recordpass.asp?RecordType=0&RecordID=2687

- **Vitiligo Fact Sheet**

  Summary: This mini-consumer health information fact sheet contains a brief description of this autoimmune skin disorder.

  Source: American Autoimmune Related Diseases Association, Inc.

  http://www.healthfinder.gov/scripts/recordpass.asp?RecordType=0&RecordID=2688

The NIH Search Utility

After browsing the references listed at the beginning of this chapter, you may want to explore the NIH Search Utility. This allows you to search for documents on over 100 selected Web sites that comprise the NIH-WEB-SPACE. Each of these servers is "crawled" and indexed on an ongoing basis. Your search will produce a list of various documents, all of which will relate in some way to vitiligo. The drawbacks of this approach are that the information is not organized by theme and that the references are often a mix of information for professionals and patients. Nevertheless, a large number of the listed Web sites provide useful background information. We can only recommend this route, therefore, for relatively rare or specific disorders, or when using highly targeted searches. To use the NIH search utility, visit the following Web page: **http://search.nih.gov/index.html**.

NORD (The National Organization of Rare Disorders, Inc.)

NORD provides an invaluable service to the public by publishing, for a nominal fee, short yet comprehensive guidelines on over 1,000 diseases. NORD primarily focuses on rare diseases that might not be covered by the previously listed sources. NORD's Web address is **www.rarediseases.org**. To see if a recent fact sheet has been published on vitiligo, simply go to the following hyperlink: **http://www.rarediseases.org/cgi-bin/nord/alphalist**. A complete guide on vitiligo can be purchased from NORD for a nominal fee.

Additional Web Sources

A number of Web sites that often link to government sites are available to the public. These can also point you in the direction of essential information. The following is a representative sample:

- AOL: **http://search.aol.com/cat.adp?id=168&layer=&from=subcats**

- drkoop.com®: **http://www.drkoop.com/conditions/ency/index.html**
- Family Village: **http://www.familyvillage.wisc.edu/specific.htm**
- Google: **http://directory.google.com/Top/Health/Conditions_and_Diseases/**
- Med Help International: **http://www.medhelp.org/HealthTopics/A.html**
- Open Directory Project: **http://dmoz.org/Health/Conditions_and_Diseases/**
- Yahoo.com: **http://dir.yahoo.com/Health/Diseases_and_Conditions/**
- WebMD®Health: **http://my.webmd.com/health_topics**

Vocabulary Builder

The material in this chapter may have contained a number of unfamiliar words. The following Vocabulary Builder introduces you to terms used in this chapter that have not been covered in the previous chapter:

Alopecia: Baldness; absence of the hair from skin areas where it normally is present. [EU]

Anemia: A reduction in the number of circulating erythrocytes or in the quantity of hemoglobin. [NIH]

Bacteria: Unicellular prokaryotic microorganisms which generally possess rigid cell walls, multiply by cell division, and exhibit three principal forms: round or coccal, rodlike or bacillary, and spiral or spirochetal. [NIH]

Biopsy: The removal and examination, usually microscopic, of tissue from the living body, performed to establish precise diagnosis. [EU]

Blister: Visible accumulations of fluid within or beneath the epidermis. [NIH]

Cataract: An opacity, partial or complete, of one or both eyes, on or in the lens or capsule, especially an opacity impairing vision or causing blindness. The many kinds of cataract are classified by their morphology (size, shape, location) or etiology (cause and time of occurrence). [EU]

Depigmentation: Removal or loss of pigment, especially melanin. [EU]

Dermatology: A medical specialty concerned with the skin, its structure, functions, diseases, and treatment. [NIH]

Dermatosis: Any skin disease, especially one not characterized by inflammation. [EU]

Dyes: Chemical substances that are used to stain and color other materials. The coloring may or may not be permanent. Dyes can also be used as therapeutic agents and test reagents in medicine and scientific research. [NIH]

Folliculitis: Inflammation of a follicle or follicles; used ordinarily in reference to hair follicles, but sometimes in relation to follicles of other kinds. [EU]

Groin: The external junctural region between the lower part of the abdomen and the thigh. [NIH]

Herpes: Any inflammatory skin disease caused by a herpesvirus and characterized by the formation of clusters of small vesicles. When used alone, the term may refer to herpes simplex or to herpes zoster. [EU]

Hormones: Chemical substances having a specific regulatory effect on the activity of a certain organ or organs. The term was originally applied to substances secreted by various endocrine glands and transported in the bloodstream to the target organs. It is sometimes extended to include those substances that are not produced by the endocrine glands but that have similar effects. [NIH]

Hyperpigmentation: Excessive pigmentation of the skin, usually as a result of increased melanization of the epidermis rather than as a result of an increased number of melanocytes. Etiology is varied and the condition may arise from exposure to light, chemicals or other substances, or from a primary metabolic imbalance. [NIH]

Hyperthyroidism: 1. excessive functional activity of the thyroid gland. 2. the abnormal condition resulting from hyperthyroidism marked by increased metabolic rate, enlargement of the thyroid gland, rapid heart rate, high blood pressure, and various secondary symptoms. [EU]

Hypothyroidism: Deficiency of thyroid activity. In adults, it is most common in women and is characterized by decrease in basal metabolic rate, tiredness and lethargy, sensitivity to cold, and menstrual disturbances. If untreated, it progresses to full-blown myxoedema. In infants, severe hypothyroidism leads to cretinism. In juveniles, the manifestations are intermediate, with less severe mental and developmental retardation and only mild symptoms of the adult form. When due to pituitary deficiency of thyrotropin secretion it is called secondary hypothyroidism. [EU]

Inflammation: A pathological process characterized by injury or destruction of tissues caused by a variety of cytologic and chemical reactions. It is usually manifested by typical signs of pain, heat, redness, swelling, and loss of function. [NIH]

Keloid: A sharply elevated, irregularly- shaped, progressively enlarging scar due to the formation of excessive amounts of collagen in the corium during connective tissue repair. [EU]

Malignant: Tending to become progressively worse and to result in death. Having the properties of anaplasia, invasion, and metastasis; said of tumours. [EU]

Melanocytes: Epidermal dendritic pigment cells which control long-term morphological color changes by alteration in their number or in the amount of pigment they produce and store in the pigment containing organelles called melanosomes. Melanophores are larger cells which do not exist in mammals. [NIH]

Melanoma: A tumour arising from the melanocytic system of the skin and other organs. When used alone the term refers to malignant melanoma. [EU]

Membrane: A thin layer of tissue which covers a surface, lines a cavity or divides a space or organ. [EU]

Nausea: An unpleasant sensation, vaguely referred to the epigastrium and abdomen, and often culminating in vomiting. [EU]

Pernicious: Tending to a fatal issue. [EU]

Photochemotherapy: Therapy using oral or topical photosensitizing agents with subsequent exposure to light. [NIH]

Phototherapy: Treatment of disease by exposure to light, especially by variously concentrated light rays or specific wavelengths. [NIH]

Pigmentation: 1. the deposition of colouring matter; the coloration or discoloration of a part by pigment. 2. coloration, especially abnormally increased coloration, by melanin. [EU]

Pityriasis: A name originally applied to a group of skin diseases characterized by the formation of fine, branny scales, but now used only with a modifier. [EU]

Proteins: Polymers of amino acids linked by peptide bonds. The specific sequence of amino acids determines the shape and function of the protein. [NIH]

Pupil: The aperture in the iris through which light passes. [NIH]

Rectal: Pertaining to the rectum (= distal portion of the large intestine). [EU]

Retina: The ten-layered nervous tissue membrane of the eye. It is continuous with the optic nerve and receives images of external objects and transmits visual impulses to the brain. Its outer surface is in contact with the choroid and the inner surface with the vitreous body. The outer-most layer is pigmented, whereas the inner nine layers are transparent. [NIH]

Suction: The removal of secretions, gas or fluid from hollow or tubular organs or cavities by means of a tube and a device that acts on negative pressure. [NIH]

Sunburn: An injury to the skin causing erythema, tenderness, and sometimes blistering and resulting from excessive exposure to the sun. The reaction is produced by the ultraviolet radiation in sunlight. [NIH]

Topical: Pertaining to a particular surface area, as a topical anti-infective applied to a certain area of the skin and affecting only the area to which it is applied. [EU]

Uveitis: An inflammation of part or all of the uvea, the middle (vascular) tunic of the eye, and commonly involving the other tunics (the sclera and cornea, and the retina). [EU]

Viruses: Minute infectious agents whose genomes are composed of DNA or RNA, but not both. They are characterized by a lack of independent metabolism and the inability to replicate outside living host cells. [NIH]

Vitiligo: A disorder consisting of areas of macular depigmentation, commonly on extensor aspects of extremities, on the face or neck, and in skin folds. Age of onset is often in young adulthood and the condition tends to progress gradually with lesions enlarging and extending until a quiescent state is reached. [NIH]

CHAPTER 2. SEEKING GUIDANCE

Overview

Some patients are comforted by the knowledge that a number of organizations dedicate their resources to helping people with vitiligo. These associations can become invaluable sources of information and advice. Many associations offer aftercare support, financial assistance, and other important services. Furthermore, healthcare research has shown that support groups often help people to better cope with their conditions.[9] In addition to support groups, your physician can be a valuable source of guidance and support. Therefore, finding a physician that can work with your unique situation is a very important aspect of your care.

In this chapter, we direct you to resources that can help you find patient organizations and medical specialists. We begin by describing how to find associations and peer groups that can help you better understand and cope with vitiligo. The chapter ends with a discussion on how to find a doctor that is right for you.

Associations and Vitiligo

As mentioned by the Agency for Healthcare Research and Quality, sometimes the emotional side of an illness can be as taxing as the physical side.[10] You may have fears or feel overwhelmed by your situation. Everyone has different ways of dealing with disease or physical injury. Your attitude, your expectations, and how well you cope with your condition can all

---

[9] Churches, synagogues, and other houses of worship might also have groups that can offer you the social support you need.

[10] This section has been adapted from http://www.ahcpr.gov/consumer/diaginf5.htm.

influence your well-being. This is true for both minor conditions and serious illnesses. For example, a study on female breast cancer survivors revealed that women who participated in support groups lived longer and experienced better quality of life when compared with women who did not participate. In the support group, women learned coping skills and had the opportunity to share their feelings with other women in the same situation.

In addition to associations or groups that your doctor might recommend, we suggest that you consider the following list (if there is a fee for an association, you may want to check with your insurance provider to find out if the cost will be covered):

- **American Autoimmune Related Diseases Association, Inc**

  Address: American Autoimmune Related Diseases Association, Inc. Michigan National Bank Building, 15475 Gratiot Avenue, Detroit, MI 48205

  Telephone: (313) 371-8600 Toll-free: (800) 598- 4668

  Fax: (313) 371-6002

  Email: aarda@aol.com

  Web Site: http://www.aarda.org

  Background: The American Autoimmune Related Diseases Association, Inc. (AARDA) is a national not-for-profit voluntary health agency dedicated to bringing a national focus to autoimmunity, a major cause of serious chronic diseases. The Association was founded for the purposes of supporting research to find a cure for autoimmune diseases and providing services to affected individuals. In addition, the Association's goals include increasing the public's awareness that autoimmunity is the cause of more than 80 serious chronic diseases; bringing national focus and collaborative effort among state and national voluntary health groups that represent autoimmune diseases; and serving as a national advocate for individuals and families affected by the physical, emotional, and financial effects of autoimmune disease. The American Autoimmune Related Diseases Association produces educational and support materials including fact sheets, brochures, pamphlets, and a newsletter entitled 'In Focus.'.

  Relevant area(s) of interest: Psoriasis, Scleroderma, Vitiligo

- **American Skin Association**

  Address: American Skin Association 150 East 58th Street, 33rd Floor, New York, NY 10155-0002

  Telephone: (212) 753-8260 Toll-free: (800) 499-7546

Fax: (212) 688-6547

Email: AmericanSkin@compuserve.com

Web Site: Non

Background: The American Skin Association (ASA) is a national nonprofit organization dedicated to building a network of lay people to achieve more effective prevention, treatment, and cure of skin disorders. ASA programs include generating support for skin research and providing information and education to the public regarding the skin and its disorders. ASA's mission is to identify, promote, and support research in biology of the skin, stimulate the transfer of advances in the field to clinical care of dermatology patients, and educate the community regarding diseases, symptoms, and care of the skin. To meet this goal, the Association engages in fundraising to support research and develops local chapters throughout the country. Information on a wide spectrum of skin disorders is available including 'Your Newborn's Skin and the Sun,' 'Ultraviolet Index: What You Need To Know,' 'Outdoor Sports and Your Skin,' and 'Proper Skin Care Can Make Gardening a Bed of Roses.' Founded in 1987, ASA also publishes 'SkinFacts,' a quarterly newsletter.

Relevant area(s) of interest: Psoriasis, Vitiligo

- **Diseases Information Clearinghouse National Institute of Arthritis and Musculoskeletal and Skin**

Address: 1 AMS Circle Bethesda, MD 20892-3675

Telephone: 301-495-4484; 877-22-NIAMS (toll-free)

Web Site: http://nih.gov/niams

Background: The National Institute of Arthritis and Musculoskeletal and Skin Diseases (NIAMS) handles inquiries on the following: arthritis, bone diseases, and skin diseases. It serves the public,patients, and health professionals by providing information, locating other information sources, creating health information materials, and participating in a national Federal database on health information.

Relevant area(s) of interest: Arthritis; Connective tissue diseases; Consumer resources; Epidermolysis bullosa; Lupus erythematosus; Musculoskeletal diseases; Osteoporosis; Paget's disease; Psoriasis; Vitiligo

- **National Foundation for Vitiligo and Pigment Disorders**

Address: National Foundation for Vitiligo and Pigment Disorders 9032 South Woemandy Lane, Centerville, OH 45458

Telephone: (937) 885-5739 Toll-free: (800) 598- 4668

Fax: (937) 885-629

Background: The National Foundation for Vitiligo and Pigment Disorders is a voluntary not-for-profit organization dedicated to educating affected individuals, family members, health care professionals, and the public about vitiligo and pigment disorders. Vitiligo is an acquired dermatological condition characterized by areas of decreased pigmentation of the skin. The lesions are usually sharply demarcated with increased coloring on the borders. Established in 1986, the National Foundation for Vitiligo and Pigment Disorders provides support to affected individuals and their families; raises funds for research; engages in patient advocacy; and provides appropriate referrals to physicians and researchers. The Foundation also provides educational and support information through its directory and various educational materials published by its parent organization, the National Vitiligo Foundation.

Relevant area(s) of interest: Vitiligo

- **National Organization for Albinism and Hypopigmentation**

  Address: National Organization for Albinism and Hypopigmentation 1530 Locust Street, Number 29, Philadelphia, PA 19102- 4415

  Telephone: (215) 545-2322 Toll-free: (800) 473- 2310

  Fax: (609) 858-4337

  Email: noah@albinism.org

  Web Site: http://www.albinism.or

  Background: The National Organization for Albinism and Hypopigmentation (NOAH) is a national voluntary not-for-profit organization for people with albinism, their families, and professionals who work with them. Established in 1982, NOAH provides a network of local chapters and contact persons; offers information, support, and appropriate referrals; and promotes public and professional education. The organization also provides networking for those with special interests related to albinism and promotes and supports research and funding that will improve diagnosis and management of albinism and hypopigmentation. Through participating in the Albinism World Alliance, NOAH networks with support groups for people with albinism in other countries and promotes development of albinism support groups throughout the world. NOAH also sponsors workshops, conferences, and outreach programs and offers a variety of educational materials including a regular newsletter, information bulletins, brochures, and information packets for libraries.

- **National Vitiligo Foundation, Inc**

  Address: National Vitiligo Foundation, Inc. 305 South Broadway, Suite 403, Tyler, TX 75702

  Telephone: (903) 531-0074 Toll-free: (800) 598- 4668

  Fax: (903) 531-9767

  Email: 73071.33@compuserve.com

  Web Site: http://www.nvfi.or

  Background: The National Vitiligo Foundation, Inc. is a voluntary not-for-profit self-help organization dedicated to providing information and support to individuals with vitiligo, a skin disorder in which pigment cells are destroyed, resulting in irregularly shaped white patches on the skin. Established in 1985, the Foundation is committed to locating, informing, and counseling affected individuals and family members; increasing public awareness and concern for affected individuals; and promoting and funding scientific and clinical research into the cause, treatment, and cure of vitiligo. The Foundation is interested in broadening the concern for people with vitiligo within the medical community and establishing a central vitiligo center and local treatment facilities across the country. In addition, the National Vitiligo Foundation promotes patient advocacy and legislation beneficial to affected individuals and engages in patient, professional, and community education. The Foundation provides a variety of informational materials including a quarterly newsletter, guidelines for physicians concerning the treatment of patients with vitiligo, fact sheets, pamphlets, and handbooks for patients, physicians, and schools.

  Relevant area(s) of interest: Vitiligo

- **XP (Xeroderma Pigmentosum) Society, Inc**

  Address:

  Telephone: (518) 851-2612 Toll-free: (800) 598- 4668

  Fax: (518) 851-2612

  Email: xps@xps.org

  Web Site: http://www.xps.or

  Background: Xeroderma Pigmentosum (XP) Society, Inc. is a national not-for-profit organization dedicated to increasing public awareness of XP and related conditions; providing direct support to individuals affected by XP and their families through information exchange and financial support; and promoting increased medical research to achieve a cure for XP. Founded in 1995, the XP Society currently has approximately 2,000 members. Xeroderma Pigmentosum is a group of rare inherited skin disorders that is characterized by a heightened reaction to sunlight (photosensitivity) with skin blistering occurring after exposure to the sun. In some cases, pain and blistering may occur immediately after contact with sunlight. Acute sunburn and persistent redness or inflammation of the skin (erythema) are also early symptoms of Xeroderma Pigmentosum. In most cases, symptoms may be apparent immediately after birth or occur within the next few years. The Society publishes a quarterly newsletter entitled 'XP Report,' distributes 'The Xeroderma Pigmentosum Handbook, A Practical Guide to Living With XP,' and sponsors 'Camp Sundown,' a yearly family summer camp for individuals affected by XP and their families.

Relevant area(s) of interest: Vitiligo

Finding More Associations

There are a number of directories that list additional medical associations that you may find useful. While not all of these directories will provide different information than what is listed above, by consulting all of them, you will have nearly exhausted all sources for patient associations.

The National Health Information Center (NHIC)

The National Health Information Center (NHIC) offers a free referral service to help people find organizations that provide information about vitiligo. For more information, see the NHIC's Web site at **http://www.health.gov/NHIC/** or contact an information specialist by calling 1-800-336-4797.

DIRLINE

A comprehensive source of information on associations is the DIRLINE database maintained by the National Library of Medicine. The database comprises some 10,000 records of organizations, research centers, and government institutes and associations which primarily focus on health and biomedicine. DIRLINE is available via the Internet at the following Web site: **http://dirline.nlm.nih.gov/**. Simply type in "vitiligo" (or a synonym) or the name of a topic, and the site will list information contained in the database on all relevant organizations.

The Combined Health Information Database

Another comprehensive source of information on healthcare associations is the Combined Health Information Database. Using the "Detailed Search" option, you will need to limit your search to "Organizations" and "vitiligo". Type the following hyperlink into your Web browser: **http://chid.nih.gov/detail/detail.html**. To find associations, use the drop boxes at the bottom of the search page where "You may refine your search by." For publication date, select "All Years." Then, select your preferred language and the format option "Organization Resource Sheet." By making these selections and typing in "vitiligo" (or synonyms) into the "For these words:" box, you will only receive results on organizations dealing with vitiligo. You should check back periodically with this database since it is updated every 3 months.

The National Organization for Rare Disorders, Inc.

The National Organization for Rare Disorders, Inc. has prepared a Web site that provides, at no charge, lists of associations organized by specific diseases. You can access this database at the following Web site: **http://www.rarediseases.org/cgi-bin/nord/searchpage**. Select the option called "Organizational Database (ODB)" and type "vitiligo" (or a synonym) in the search box.

Online Support Groups

In addition to support groups, commercial Internet service providers offer forums and chat rooms for people with different illnesses and conditions. WebMD®, for example, offers such a service at their Web site: **http://boards.webmd.com/roundtable**. These online self-help communities can help you connect with a network of people whose concerns are similar to yours. Online support groups are places where people can talk informally. If you read about a novel approach, consult with your doctor or other healthcare providers, as the treatments or discoveries you hear about may not be scientifically proven to be safe and effective. The following Internet sites may be of particular interest:

- **Med Help International**
  http://www.medhelp.org/HealthTopics/Vitiligo.html

- **Vitiligo Support**
  http://www.vitiligosupport.com

- **Patient UK**
  http://www.patient.co.uk/illness/v/vitiligo.htm

Finding Doctors

One of the most important aspects of your treatment will be the relationship between you and your doctor or specialist. All patients with vitiligo must go through the process of selecting a physician. While this process will vary from person to person, the Agency for Healthcare Research and Quality makes a number of suggestions, including the following:[11]

- If you are in a managed care plan, check the plan's list of doctors first.

- Ask doctors or other health professionals who work with doctors, such as hospital nurses, for referrals.

- Call a hospital's doctor referral service, but keep in mind that these services usually refer you to doctors on staff at that particular hospital. The services do not have information on the quality of care that these doctors provide.

- Some local medical societies offer lists of member doctors. Again, these lists do not have information on the quality of care that these doctors provide.

Additional steps you can take to locate doctors include the following:

- Check with the associations listed earlier in this chapter.

- Information on doctors in some states is available on the Internet at **http://www.docboard.org**. This Web site is run by "Administrators in Medicine," a group of state medical board directors.

- The American Board of Medical Specialties can tell you if your doctor is board certified. "Certified" means that the doctor has completed a training program in a specialty and has passed an exam, or "board," to assess his or her knowledge, skills, and experience to provide quality patient care in that specialty. Primary care doctors may also be certified as specialists. The AMBS Web site is located at

---

[11] This section is adapted from the AHRQ: www.ahrq.gov/consumer/qntascii/qntdr.htm.

http://www.abms.org/newsearch.asp.[12] You can also contact the ABMS by phone at 1-866-ASK-ABMS.

- You can call the American Medical Association (AMA) at 800-665-2882 for information on training, specialties, and board certification for many licensed doctors in the United States. This information also can be found in "Physician Select" at the AMA's Web site: **http://www.ama-assn.org/aps/amahg.htm.**

If the previous sources did not meet your needs, you may want to log on to the Web site of the National Organization for Rare Disorders (NORD) at **http://www.rarediseases.org/**. NORD maintains a database of doctors with expertise in various rare diseases. The Metabolic Information Network (MIN), 800-945-2188, also maintains a database of physicians with expertise in various metabolic diseases.

Finding a Dermatologist

To find a dermatologist in your area, you can use the "Find a Dermatologist" search engine provided by the American Academy of Dermatology. With a membership of 13,000, the American Academy of Dermatology represents virtually all practicing dermatologists in the United States and Canada. Type the following Web address into your browser to begin your search: **http://www.aad.org/DermSearch/index.html**. To search for dermatologists by U.S. state, enter your state into the search box and click "Search." To search for dermatologists practicing outside the U.S., select "international members." Enter your country and click the "Search" button.

Selecting Your Doctor[3]

When you have compiled a list of prospective doctors, call each of their offices. First, ask if the doctor accepts your health insurance plan and if he or she is taking new patients. If the doctor is not covered by your plan, ask yourself if you are prepared to pay the extra costs. The next step is to schedule a visit with your chosen physician. During the first visit you will have the opportunity to evaluate your doctor and to find out if you feel comfortable with him or her. Ask yourself, did the doctor:

---

[12] While board certification is a good measure of a doctor's knowledge, it is possible to receive quality care from doctors who are not board certified.
[13] This section has been adapted from the AHRQ: www.ahrq.gov/consumer/qntascii/qntdr.htm.

- Give me a chance to ask questions about vitiligo?
- Really listen to my questions?
- Answer in terms I understood?
- Show respect for me?
- Ask me questions?
- Make me feel comfortable?
- Address the health problem(s) I came with?
- Ask me my preferences about different kinds of treatments for vitiligo?
- Spend enough time with me?

Trust your instincts when deciding if the doctor is right for you. But remember, it might take time for the relationship to develop. It takes more than one visit for you and your doctor to get to know each other.

Working with Your Doctor[14]

Research has shown that patients who have good relationships with their doctors tend to be more satisfied with their care and have better results. Here are some tips to help you and your doctor become partners:

- You know important things about your symptoms and your health history. Tell your doctor what you think he or she needs to know.
- It is important to tell your doctor personal information, even if it makes you feel embarrassed or uncomfortable.
- Bring a "health history" list with you (and keep it up to date).
- Always bring any medications you are currently taking with you to the appointment, or you can bring a list of your medications including dosage and frequency information. Talk about any allergies or reactions you have had to your medications.
- Tell your doctor about any natural or alternative medicines you are taking.
- Bring other medical information, such as x-ray films, test results, and medical records.

---

14 This section has been adapted from the AHRQ:
www.ahrq.gov/consumer/qntascii/qntdr.htm.

- Ask questions. If you don't, your doctor will assume that you understood everything that was said.

- Write down your questions before your visit. List the most important ones first to make sure that they are addressed.

- Consider bringing a friend with you to the appointment to help you ask questions. This person can also help you understand and/or remember the answers.

- Ask your doctor to draw pictures if you think that this would help you understand.

- Take notes. Some doctors do not mind if you bring a tape recorder to help you remember things, but always ask first.

- Let your doctor know if you need more time. If there is not time that day, perhaps you can speak to a nurse or physician assistant on staff or schedule a telephone appointment.

- Take information home. Ask for written instructions. Your doctor may also have brochures and audio and videotapes that can help you.

- After leaving the doctor's office, take responsibility for your care. If you have questions, call. If your symptoms get worse or if you have problems with your medication, call. If you had tests and do not hear from your doctor, call for your test results. If your doctor recommended that you have certain tests, schedule an appointment to get them done. If your doctor said you should see an additional specialist, make an appointment.

By following these steps, you will enhance the relationship you will have with your physician.

Broader Health-Related Resources

In addition to the references above, the NIH has set up guidance Web sites that can help patients find healthcare professionals. These include:[15]

- Caregivers:
  http://www.nlm.nih.gov/medlineplus/caregivers.html

- Choosing a Doctor or Healthcare Service:
  http://www.nlm.nih.gov/medlineplus/choosingadoctororhealthcareserv ice.html

---

[15] You can access this information at:
http://www.nlm.nih.gov/medlineplus/healthsystem.html.

- Hospitals and Health Facilities:
  http://www.nlm.nih.gov/medlineplus/healthfacilities.html

Vocabulary Builder

The following vocabulary builder provides definitions of words used in this chapter that have not been defined in previous chapters:

Albinism: General term for a number of inherited defects of amino acid metabolism in which there is a deficiency or absence of pigment in the eyes, skin, or hair. [NIH]

Autoimmunity: Process whereby the immune system reacts against the body's own tissues. Autoimmunity may produce or be caused by autoimmune diseases. [NIH]

Hypopigmentation: A condition caused by a deficiency in melanin formation or a loss of pre-existing melanin or melanocytes. It can be complete or partial and may result from trauma, inflammation, and certain infections. [NIH]

Lesion: Any pathological or traumatic discontinuity of tissue or loss of function of a part. [EU]

Lupus: A form of cutaneous tuberculosis. It is seen predominantly in women and typically involves the nasal, buccal, and conjunctival mucosa. [NIH]

Osteoporosis: Reduction in the amount of bone mass, leading to fractures after minimal trauma. [EU]

Photosensitivity: An abnormal cutaneous response involving the interaction between photosensitizing substances and sunlight or filtered or artificial light at wavelengths of 280-400 mm. There are two main types : photoallergy and photoxicity. [EU]

Psoriasis: A common genetically determined, chronic, inflammatory skin disease characterized by rounded erythematous, dry, scaling patches. The lesions have a predilection for nails, scalp, genitalia, extensor surfaces, and the lumbosacral region. Accelerated epidermopoiesis is considered to be the fundamental pathologic feature in psoriasis. [NIH]

Spectrum: A charted band of wavelengths of electromagnetic vibrations obtained by refraction and diffraction. By extension, a measurable range of activity, such as the range of bacteria affected by an antibiotic (antibacterial s.) or the complete range of manifestations of a disease. [EU]

PART II: ADDITIONAL RESOURCES AND ADVANCED MATERIAL

ABOUT PART II

In Part II, we introduce you to additional resources and advanced research on vitiligo. All too often, patients who conduct their own research are overwhelmed by the difficulty in finding and organizing information. The purpose of the following chapters is to provide you an organized and structured format to help you find additional information resources on vitiligo. In Part II, as in Part I, our objective is not to interpret the latest advances on vitiligo or render an opinion. Rather, our goal is to give you access to original research and to increase your awareness of sources you may not have already considered. In this way, you will come across the advanced materials often referred to in pamphlets, books, or other general works. Once again, some of this material is technical in nature, so consultation with a professional familiar with vitiligo is suggested.

CHAPTER 3. STUDIES ON VITILIGO

Overview

Every year, academic studies are published on vitiligo or related conditions. Broadly speaking, there are two types of studies. The first are peer reviewed. Generally, the content of these studies has been reviewed by scientists or physicians. Peer-reviewed studies are typically published in scientific journals and are usually available at medical libraries. The second type of studies is non-peer reviewed. These works include summary articles that do not use or report scientific results. These often appear in the popular press, newsletters, or similar periodicals.

In this chapter, we will show you how to locate peer-reviewed references and studies on vitiligo. We will begin by discussing research that has been summarized and is free to view by the public via the Internet. We then show you how to generate a bibliography on vitiligo and teach you how to keep current on new studies as they are published or undertaken by the scientific community.

The Combined Health Information Database

The Combined Health Information Database summarizes studies across numerous federal agencies. To limit your investigation to research studies and vitiligo, you will need to use the advanced search options. First, go to **http://chid.nih.gov/index.html**. From there, select the "Detailed Search" option (or go directly to that page with the following hyperlink: **http://chid.nih.gov/detail/detail.html**). The trick in extracting studies is found in the drop boxes at the bottom of the search page where "You may refine your search by." Select the dates and language you prefer, and the format option "Journal Article." At the top of the search form, select the number of records you would like to see (we recommend 100) and check the box to display "whole records." We recommend that you type in "vitiligo" (or synonyms) into the "For these words:" box. Consider using the option "anywhere in record" to make your search as broad as possible. If you want to limit the search to only a particular field, such as the title of the journal, then select this option in the "Search in these fields" drop box. The following is a sample of what you can expect from this type of search:

- **Psychologic Effects of Vitiligo: A Critical Incident Analysis**

  Source: Journal of the American Academy of Dermatology. 35:895-898; December 1996.

  Summary: This journal article for health professionals describes a study that combined qualitative and quantitative methods in a large patient group to provide an indication of the extent of the social and psychological consequences of vitiligo. A circular was enclosed with the quarterly Newsletter of the Vitiligo Society inviting members to participate in the study. A usable sample of 614 members of the U.K. Vitiligo Society was obtained. Participants completed a questionnaire that included the 12-item version of the General Health Questionnaire (GHQ) and an open-ended question concerning the effects of the disease on their life. Results indicate that 35 percent of the respondents scored above the threshold on the GHQ. Analysis of the qualitative data indicate that vitiligo affected lives in a variety of ways consistent with perceived stigma and that some categories of response, such as avoidance of activities and negative reactions by others, were associated with higher GHQ scores. Results suggest that many persons with vitiligo show indications of significant distress that are related to specific types of social encounters and emotional disturbance. 29 references and 2 tables. (AA-M).

- **Cytomegalovirus DNA Identified in Skin Biopsy Specimens of Patients with Vitiligo**

  Source: Journal of the American Academy of Dermatology. 35:21-26; July 1996.

  Summary: This study determined the presence or absence of viral genomes in the depigmented and uninvolved skin of patients with vitiligo. Researchers used a polymerase chain reaction assay to detect viral genomes in paraffinembedded skin biopsy specimens. Twenty-nine patients with vitiligo and 22 control subjects participated. Biopsy specimens were screened in a blinded fashion for a panel of DNA and RNA viruses included herpes simplex, varicella-zoster, cytomegalovirus

(CMV), Epstein-Barr, HIV, and human T-cell lymphotropic virus. Results show that CMV DNA was identified in 38 percent of the patients studied. Twenty-one percent had indeterminate results. Results in all control subjects were negative. Polymerase chain reaction screening for identification of other viral genomes was negative. Although not statistically significant, data trends suggested a correlation between the presence of CMV DNA in biopsy specimens and active vitiligo of relatively brief duration. In addition, CMV-positive patients had a statistically significant increased frequency of other concurrent autoimmune diseases. The results suggest that vitiligo may indeed by triggered by a viral infection in select patients. 3 tables, 52 references. (AA-M).

- **Skin Disorders in IBD**

  Source: Foundation Focus. p. 10-11. April 1994.

  Contact: Available from Crohn's and Colitis Foundation of America, Inc. 386 Park Avenue South, 17th Floor, New York, NY 10016-8804. (800) 343-3637 or (800) 932-2423 or (212) 685-3440.

  Summary: In this newsletter article, the author reviews the various skin disorders seen in inflammatory bowel disease (IBD) and provides information about their causes and treatment. The author notes that up to one-fourth of persons with Crohn's disease or ulcerative colitis may have skin involvement as part of their disease. The article addresses direct extensions of IBD, including fissures and fistulas, metastatic Crohn's disease, and oral Crohn's disease; reactions to IBD, including erythema nodosum, pyoderma gangrenosum, aphthous ulcerations, vasculitis, and pyoderma vegetans; nutritional deficiencies, notably acrodermatitis enteropathica; complications of drug therapy; and miscellaneous problems, including epidermolysis bullosa, vitiligo, psoriasis, and clubbing.

- **Superficial Fungal Infection of the Skin: Where and How It Appears Help Determine Therapy**

  Source: Postgraduate Medicine. 109(1): 117-120,123-126,131-132. January 2001.

  Summary: This journal article provides health professionals with information on the features, diagnosis, and management of tinea pedis, tinea corporis, tinea cruris, tinea versicolor, tinea capitis, tinea faciei, tinea manuum, cutaneous candidiasis, and onychomycosis. Tinea pedis, the most common fungal infection of the skin, involves the plantar surface and interdigital spaces of the foot and can include inflammatory and noninflammatory lesions. Differential diagnosis of tinea pedis includes acrodermatitis continua, candidiasis, contact dermatitis, eczema, erythrasma, psoriasis, pustular bacterids, pyoderma, and secondary syphilis. Tinea pedis usually responds to topical agents such as econazole nitrate, ketoconazole, and terbinafine hydrochloride. Tinea corporis, commonly referred to as ringworm of the body, is dermatophytosis of the glabrous skin of the trunk and extremities. This condition typically develops after inappropriate topical corticosteroid therapy. Treatment involves topical therapy. Tinea cruris, or jock itch, is a dermatophytosis of the proximal medial thigh and buttock. Differential diagnosis includes mechanical intertrigo and candidiasis. Treatment involves topical therapy. Tinea versicolor, or pityriasis versicolor, is typically found in regions of the body that have sebaceous glands. The characteristic finding is skin depigmentation. Differential diagnosis includes vitiligo, tinea corporis, pityriasis rosea, pityriasis alba, and secondary syphilis. Topical therapies such as terbinafine, econazole, ketoconazole, and selenium sulfide lotion or shampoo are effective topical therapies. Tinea capitis, which is a dermatophytic infection of the head and scalp, can have a range of clinical presentations. Differential diagnosis includes seborrheic dermatitis, dandruff, scalp psoriasis, atopic dermatitis, and alopecia areata. An oral agent such as griseofulvin is usually needed to successfully treat this condition. Tinea faciei is dermatophytosis of the nonbearded areas of the face. This infection responds to topical therapy. Tinea manuum, an unusual dermatophytic infection of the interdigital and palmar surfaces, may coexist with other fungal infections. Differential diagnosis includes pompholyx, eczema, secondary syphilis, and callus formation. Although the condition responds to topical therapy, it may recur if untreated onychomycosis is present. Cutaneous candidiasis, a skin infection caused by Candida albicans and other species, often presents with erythema, cracking, or maceration. Topical agents commonly used to treat this condition include nystatin, ketoconazole, miconazole nitrate, and clotrimazole. Onychomycosis, a fungal infection of the nail unit, has a wide variety of clinical presentations. Differential diagnosis includes psoriasis, lichen planus, alopecia areata, subungual tumors and warts, and bacterial infections. Oral agents are more successful than topical agents. The article also discusses the topical and systemic agents used to treat cutaneous fungal infections. Topical agents include imidazoles, allylamines, and polyenes. Systemic agents include griseofulvin, ketoconazole, itraconazole, terbinafine, and fluconazole. 16 figures, 2 tables, and 21 references.

- **Guidelines of Care for Vitiligo**

  Source: Journal of the American Academy of Dermatology. 35(4):620-626; October 1996.

  Summary: This journal article for health professionals presents guidelines of care for vitiligo. This condition is defined, and the rationale for the guidelines is presented. Diagnostic criteria are outlined, including clinical criteria and physical examination findings. Tests that may be useful in the diagnosis of vitiligo are highlighted. Recommendations concerning the treatment of vitiligo are presented, focusing on topical and oral psoralen photochemotherapy, heliotherapy, topical corticosteroid therapy, depigmentation, adjunctive therapy, surgery, and evolving therapies. 30 references.

Federally-Funded Research on Vitiligo

The U.S. Government supports a variety of research studies relating to vitiligo and associated conditions. These studies are tracked by the Office of Extramural Research at the National Institutes of Health.[16] CRISP (Computerized Retrieval of Information on Scientific Projects) is a searchable database of federally-funded biomedical research projects conducted at universities, hospitals, and other institutions. Visit the CRISP Web site at **http://commons.cit.nih.gov/crisp3/CRISP.Generate_Ticket**. You can perform targeted searches by various criteria including geography, date, as well as topics related to vitiligo and related conditions.

For most of the studies, the agencies reporting into CRISP provide summaries or abstracts. As opposed to clinical trial research using patients, many federally-funded studies use animals or simulated models to explore vitiligo and related conditions. In some cases, therefore, it may be difficult to understand how some basic or fundamental research could eventually translate into medical practice. The following sample is typical of the type of information found when searching the CRISP database for vitiligo:

---

[16] Healthcare projects are funded by the National Institutes of Health (NIH), Substance Abuse and Mental Health Services (SAMHSA), Health Resources and Services Administration (HRSA), Food and Drug Administration (FDA), Centers for Disease Control and Prevention (CDCP), Agency for Healthcare Research and Quality (AHRQ), and Office of Assistant Secretary of Health (OASH).

- **Project Title: IGF-1 Apoptotic Defenses in Melanocytes and Vitiligo**

Principal Investigator & Institution: Morelli, Joseph G.; Dermatology; University of Colorado Hlth Sciences Ctr 4200 E 9Th Ave Denver, Co 80262

Timing: Fiscal Year 2000; Project Start 1-JUN-2000; Project End 1-MAY-2003

Summary: Vitiligo affects 1 percent of the population worldwide. This very common skin affliction is of great significance among dark skinned people in the United States and worldwide. In many countries and societies people with vitiligo are treated as outcasts. We propose that the defenses of melanocytes against cell death are overcome in vitiligo, and must be restored during vitiligo repigmentation. We hypothesize that Insulin-like Growth Factor 1 (IGF-1) is a critical mediator of melanocyte function, stimulating melanocyte movement and proliferation and promoting melanocyte survival by maintaining anti-apoptotic defenses. This proposal will define the IGF-1 anti-apoptotic defenses of melanocytes. Specific Aim 1 will demonstrate that IGF-1 maintains the resistance of human melanocytes to apoptosis and will determine which anti-apoptotic proteins are controlled by IGF-1. Specific Aim 2 will determine which of these IFG-1 effects are mediated through the Ras signaling pathway. Specific Aim 3 will determine whether IGF-1 dependent anti-apoptotic defenses are mediated through PI3K or AKT/PBK. Specific Aim 4 will determine whether intergrin receptors and the IGF-1 receptor act synergistically to control anti-apoptotic defenses in melanocytes. These project is innovative because it: i). Applies modern knowledge of the molecular control of apoptosis and cell death to the study of melanocyte survival, a fundamental biologic feature relevant to human vitiligo, and ii) focuses attention on the role of IGF-1 in melanocyte biology. IGF-1 is a powerful mediator of melanocyte function and mediates crucial survival mechanism in other types of cells. The experiments proposed in this RO3 grant will provide the preliminary data for a future RO1 on IGF-1 as a survival factor in vitiligo. The detailed mechanistic studies of IGF-1 control of melanocyte survival will provide a proper basis for questions concerning the relative role of IGF-1 in melanocyte destruction in vitiligo, and of melanocyte survival during repigmentation of vitiligo.

Website: http://commons.cit.nih.gov/crisp3/CRISP.Generate_Ticket

- **Project Title: Mapping of Vitiligo Susceptibility Genes**

Principal Investigator & Institution: Spritz, Richard A.; Professor and Director; Biochem & Molecular Genetics; University of Colorado Hlth Sciences Ctr 4200 E 9Th Ave Denver, Co 80262

Timing: Fiscal Year 2000; Project Start 1-SEP-1999; Project End 1-AUG-2003

Summary: Generalized vitiligo is a common, non-contagious disorder, characterized by progressive patchy loss of pigmentation of the skin, overlying hair, oral mucosa, and occasionally eyes, due to progressive loss of pigment forming melanocytes in the affected areas Vitiligo is thought to be autoimmune in origin, and frequently is associated with other autoimmune disorders. The prevalence of vitiligo is approximately 0.1 to 0.3 percent in different ethnic or racial groups. Vitiligo is most significant in dark-skinned populations, for its pigmentary disfigurement produces social stigmatization and is often confused with leprosy or other socially terrifying infectious diseases. But it can be a devastating disorder to those affected in any population. In preparation for this study, we conducted a survey of vitiligo patients in the United Kingdom, the largest ever done, thereby ascertaining a large cohort of families with vitiligo. These data were consistent with other studies in suggesting a total risk to first-degree relative of probands of about 7%. Further, one or more susceptibility loci appears to account for an apparent autosomal dominant inheritance of vitiligo. Further, one or more susceptibility loci appears to account for an apparent autosomal dominant inheritance of vitiligo in a fraction (approximately 8%) of families. However, the major gene(s) in these families does not account for the total increased risk for vitiligo in relatives, suggesting that susceptibility alleles with lower penetrance at the same or different loci are important in other families. These results suggest a mixed model for the inheritance of vitiligo, which has also been reported for many other complex disorders. The proposed studies will combine the UK vitiligo family cohort with a similarly sized vitiligo family cohort in the USA. Utilizing these resources, and 400 polymorphic markers spaced at approximately 10 cM intervals throughout the genome, we proposed a two-phased approach to mapping vitiligo susceptibility loci. The specific aims are: 1) Map autosomal dominant vitiligo susceptibility loci by parametric linkage analysis in families with 4 or more affected relatives; and (2) map other vitiligo susceptibility loci by parametric linkage analysis in families with 4 or more affected relatives; and (2) map other susceptibility genes using non-parametric linkage analysis in affected sib pairs. This rational and comprehensive approach will provide the greatest likelihood of mapping vitiligo susceptibility loci, thereby accelerating the identification, and the molecular, cellular, clinical, and epidemiological characterization, of the disease genes.

Website: http://commons.cit.nih.gov/crisp3/CRISP.Generate_Ticket

- **Project Title: Phenols/Catechols in Occupational/Contact Vitiligo Skin**

Principal Investigator & Institution: Boissy, Raymond E.; Associate Professor; Dermatology; University of Cincinnati 2624 Clifton Ave Cincinnati, Oh 45221

Timing: Fiscal Year 2000; Project Start 1-AUG-2000; Project End 1-JUL-2003

Summary: Complexion coloration is essential to ones health, self-image, and thus overall wellness, both physically and psychologically. Cutaneous pigmentation protects a person from various environmental assaults, like ultraviolet light, as well as potential cellular injury, that can cause cancer and aging of the skin. Loss of skin pigmentation can result in cancer, aging, and compromised immunity of the skin as well as psychological and social problems of self- esteem and personal interactions. Occupational/contact vitiligo is a disease that results in the loss of cutaneous pigmentation. This form of vitiligo occurs relatively frequently in individuals exposed to phenolic/catecholic derivatives primarily in the work place. This disease can be financially and socially devastating for the individual, in addition to it compromising the productivity in the workplace. The general goal of this proposal is to assess the pathological effects of phenolic and catecholic derivatives on melanocytes. These prevalent chemical toxins are responsible for the development of occupational/contact vitiligo in the skin of some individuals exposed to these environmental agents in the workplace. Specifically, we propose to assess the relative cytotoxicity, the interaction with tyrosinase, and the generation of toxic free radical products within melanocytes exposed to various phenolic and catecholic derivatives. In this assessment, we will determine whether melanocytes from all patients with vitiligo, patients with the occupational/contact form of vitiligo, family members of patients with vitiligo, and/or a subset of the population in general, are more sensitive to cytotoxicity by these phenolic/catecholic derivatives. In addition, we will assess [1] genes that are differentially expressed and [2] regulators of apoptosis in cells treated with phenolic/catecholic derivatives. In addition, we will determine whether the response of these molecules is altered in vitiligo melanocytes demonstrated to be more susceptible to cytotoxicity. Finally, we will assess the effectiveness of various antioxidants, especially catalase, in dampening the cytotoxic effect of phenolic/catecholic derivatives using cultured melanocytes, organotypic cultures of human skin, and a guinea pig model.

Website: http://commons.cit.nih.gov/crisp3/CRISP.Generate_Ticket

- **Project Title: R METHUSCF in Patients w/ Vitiligo**

Principal Investigator & Institution: Pandya, Amit G.; ; University of Texas Sw Med Ctr/Dallas Southwestern Medical Ctr/Dallas Dallas, Tx 75390

Timing: Fiscal Year 2000

Summary: This abstract is not available.

Website: http://commons.cit.nih.gov/crisp3/CRISP.Generate_Ticket

- **Project Title: Role of Melanocyte Defect in Smyth Line Vitiligo**

Principal Investigator & Institution: Erf, Gisela F.; Assistant Professor; Poultry Science; University of Arkansas at Fayetteville Administration Bldg 422 Fayetteville, Ar 72701

Timing: Fiscal Year 2001; Project Start 1-JUL-2001; Project End 0-JUN-2004

Summary: (provided by applicant): Vitiligo is a common acquired hypopigmentary disorder characterized by a loss of epidermal melanocytes. Although the pathogenesis of vitiligo is still poorly understood, evidence suggests that in many cases vitiligo is an autoimmune disorder and melanocyte loss is the result of an immunological response. The mutant Smyth line chicken is an accepted animal model for autoimmune vitiligo. Chickens from this line develop a spontaneous, vitiligo-like, postnatal loss of melanin producing pigment cells (melanocytes) in feather and choroidal tissue between 6 and 14 weeks of age. Like many autoimmune diseases, SL vitiligo is a multifactorial disorder, involving an inherent melanocyte defect, an immune system component, and an environmental component. Studies examining the basic defect manifested within the SL melanocyte describe the presence of a competent pigment system at hatch. Prior to visible signs of vitiligo, the earliest abnormality detected within SL melanocytes are irregularly shaped melanosomes containing pigmented membrane extensions, hyperactive melanization, and selective autophagocytosis of melanosomes. These aberrant processes precede the degeneration of SL melanocytes in vivo and in vitro but are not sufficient to cause the expression of vitiligo without a functioning immune system. Mechanisms underlying the dysfunction, progressive degeneration, and eventually, immune recognition and destruction of SL melanocytes are poorly understood. It is the goal of this proposal to study the mechanism by which the local and internal environment of the vitiliginous SL melanocyte contributes to and/or results in the degeneration of melanocytes and the development of autoimmune vitiligo. Specifically, we propose to investigate the role of oxidative stress, antioxidant capacity, inflammatory mediators and immunofunctional activities of melanocytes in the degeneration/survival of melanocytes in vivo and in vitro. These studies will be carried out using feather tissue and melanocyte cultures from SL chickens that are highly susceptible to the development of vitiligo, parental BL chickens that are susceptible to the development of vitiligo but rarely express vitiligo, and LBL chickens that are vitiligo resistant. The knowledge that will be gained from these studies regarding the underlying mechanism of the SL melanocyte's inherent susceptibility for degeneration and autoimmune destruction. may open up new venues for treatment and prevention of this disorder.

Website: http://commons.cit.nih.gov/crisp3/CRISP.Generate_Ticket

- **Project Title: Serological Expression Analysis of Vitiligo and Alopecia**

Principal Investigator & Institution: Setaluri, Vijayasaradhi; Associate Professor; Dermatology; Wake Forest University Reynolda Sta Winston-Salem, Nc 27109

Timing: Fiscal Year 2000; Project Start 1-SEP-2000; Project End 1-AUG-2002

Summary: (Taken from the application): Autoimmune reactions to components of skin and its appendages produce a spectrum of skin diseases. Vitiligo, characterized by partial or complete loss of skin pigmentation and alopecia areata, a chronic inflammatory hair disorder are two such diseases. Interestingly, while certain autoimmune skin disorders such as bullous diseases result from reactions limited to specific components of skin, vitiligo and alopecia often manifest in association with other autoimmune diseases. This suggests that immune tolerance to self-antigens on pigment producing melanocytes and cells in the hair follicles is broken relatively easily. The molecular identity of these antigens and the role of humoral vs. cellular immune responses in the pathogenesis of these diseases remain unknown. Biochemical and immunocytochemical techniques employed to identify antigens recognized by autoantibodies in the sera of patients have failed to yield definitive knowledge of target antigens in these disorders. Similarly, methodological limitations in analyzing and characterizing T lymphocytes in vitro have precluded extensive studies on the role of T cells in the pathogenesis of vitiligo and alopecia. Recent developments in the field of human tumor immunology provide an opportunity to overcome these limitations on molecular identification of targets for immune responses in autoimmune skin disorders. First, it has been demonstrated that screening cDNA expression libraries with serum antibodies from cancer patients can be used to identify antigen targets for humoral responses. Second, this screening method, termed SEREX, also allows identification of antigens recognized by cytotoxic CD8 T cells in patients with cancer. Together with recent studies that showed the presence of HLA class II-restricted CD4 T cells to tumor antigen recognized by CD8 cells, these observations from SEREX analysis reinforce the concept of simultaneous presentation of self-antigens to humoral and cellular immune systems. This raises the possibility that SEREX analysis with sera from patients with autoimmune skin disorders could allow identification of tissue-specific antigens recognized by antibodies and T cells. Molecular identification of the array of antigens targeted for immune response in these diseases will help delineate mechanisms of their pathogenesis. We propose to generate cDNA expression libraries from pooled cultures of neonatal melanocytes obtained from different racial backgrounds and pooled hair follicles microdissected from normal scalp biopsies. These expression libraries will provide a source of unlimited supply of tissue-specific gene products to begin dissecting immune responses by SEREX analysis. It is expected that such analysis will allow identification of targets for both antibody and T cell responses in vitiligo and alopecia areata.

Website: http://commons.cit.nih.gov/crisp3/CRISP.Generate_Ticket

- **Project Title: Conference--Pigment Cell Research**

Principal Investigator & Institution: King, Richard A.; Professor; Medicine; University of Minnesota Twin Cities Twin Cities Minneapolis, Mn 55455

Timing: Fiscal Year 2001; Project Start 9-JUL-2001; Project End 8-JUL-2002

Summary: (Taken from the applicant's abstract): The PanAmerican Society for Pigment Cell Research (PASPCR) was established in 1987 for scientists and physicians from North, Central and South America who study the normal and abnormal biology of melanogenesis and the melanocyte. The PASPCR was started at the beginning of a decade in biological research. Molecular biology has become widely applied and the methods and techniques for investigation have changed dramatically. It is now time to expand the horizon of the society, by bringing important and new disciplines within its vision. The 2001 10th Annual Meeting has been organized with symposia to bring new areas and new approaches to the study of the pigment cell. This meeting will be held in Minneapolis on June 14-17, 2001. The theme of this meeting will be New Approaches to the Pigment Cell. The overall objectives of the meeting are to expand ideas, approaches and collaborations for members of the society by bringing together experts from other disciplines of science who work in areas that are or should be relevant to pigment cell research and associated diseases such as melanoma, albinism and vitiligo. The Specific

Aims of the proposed efforts are: 1. To provide partial support the travel and meeting expenses for 15 Invited Speakers for five symposia during the 10th annual meeting of the PASPCR. These speakers are internationally recognized as leaders in their field, and, except for two, and not members of the PASPCR. 2. To provide partial support for room, poster and audiovisual expenses for the 10th annual meeting of the PASPCR.

Website: http://commons.cit.nih.gov/crisp3/CRISP.Generate_Ticket

- **Project Title: Cutaneous Biology of Nitric Oxide**

Principal Investigator & Institution: Lerner, Ethan A.; Associate Professor; Massachusetts General Hospital 55 Fruit St Boston, Ma 02114

Timing: Fiscal Year 2000; Project Start 0-SEP-1998; Project End 1-AUG-2003

Summary: It is proposed that nitric oxide (NO) is a critical messenger and effector molecule in skin physiology and homeostasis and that altered levels of NO in the skin cause disease. The goal of the proposal is to define the role of NO in skin with an emphasis towards determining the functional effects of this gas. Human, but not murine, keratinocytes have been demonstrated to have the capacity to express inducible form of nitric oxide synthase (iNOS) and produce NO. This critical difference between mice and men may explain why mice do not develop cutaneous eruptions analogous to those found in humans. Transgenic mice in which NOS is targeted to the skin mimic are shown here to develop phenotype found in human conditions. In conventional mice, iNOS is expressed in Langerhans cells (LC). NO is also produced by the LC-like cell line XS-52. NO produced in LC may affect LC function and, as NO is freely diffusible across cell membranes, it has the capacity to affect adjacent cells in the epidermis. Toxic effects of NO on melanocytes and keratinocytes suggest that NO may be an effector molecules in a number of skin conditions, including post-inflammatory hypo-pigmentation, vitiligo, graft versus host disease (GVH), scleroderma and the often fatal process, toxic epidermal necrolysis (TEN). In the proposed studies, purified LC will be evaluated for the production of iNOS using RT-PCR and measurement of NO using the Griess reaction and the conversion of radioactive L-arginine to citrulline. The effects of selected cytokines in the regulation of NOS will be examined. The effects of NO on XS-52 cells themselves will be studied. The mechanism of NO-induced killing of melanocytes and keratinocytes will be examined in co-culture experiments with XS-52 cells and via incubation with NO donors. Transgenic mice in which NOS expression is targeted to the epidermis have been produced, phenotypically develop white hair and histopathologically, scleroderma. These animals will be characterized further. Mice expressing NOS under the control of an inducible promoter will be generated. The transgenic mice will be tested as models for disorders of pigmentation, antigen presentation, scleroderma, TEN and GVH. These results have the potential to lead to novel therapeutic strategies for the treatment of human disease.

Website: http://commons.cit.nih.gov/crisp3/CRISP.Generate_Ticket

- **Project Title: Cytotoxic Mechanisms in Cutaneous Disease**

Principal Investigator & Institution: Norris, David A.; Professor; Dermatology; University of Colorado Hlth Sciences Ctr 4200 E 9Th Ave Denver, Co 80262

Timing: Fiscal Year 2000; Project Start 1-JAN-1980; Project End 1-AUG-2002

Summary: This is a request for an additional five years of funding for "Cytotoxic Mechanisms in Cutaneous Disease" which has been funded to sixteen years to study the mechanisms of immunologic damage to keratinocytes and melanocytes, a central component in important skin diseases such as photosensitive lupus erythematosus, vitiligo, erythema multiforme, toxic epidermal necrolysis and lichen planus. We have found that the epidermis is intrinsically resistant to immunologic cytotoxicity, due in large part to resistance of basal keratinocytes and melanocytes to apoptosis induced by immunologic triggers. We hypothesize that this resistance to apoptosis in undifferentiated keratinocytes and melanocytes is maintained by "survival" signals provided by growth factor activation of receptors and by extracellular matrix activating cell surface integrins. We propose to test the effect of growth factor and integrin blockade on the susceptibility of melanocytes and keratinocytes to induction of apoptosis by ultraviolet radiation (UVR), ionophore, anti-Fas, and cytokines. Using combinations of blocking, rescue and transfection experiments, we will verify that survival signals in melanocytes and keratinocytes are transmitted through ras activation, and directly regulate expression of important proteins which control apoptosis, such as bc1-2, and perhaps bc1-x, Bax and Bad. We will also study regulation of these important proteins following nuclear translocation of p53, and important trigger of apoptosis induced by UVR. This proposal addresses the molecular and cellular biology of a fundamental characteristic of the basal layer of the epidermis: its intrinsic resistance to immunologic cytotoxicity. Although these anti- apoptotic defenses protect the skin from unwanted effects of inflammation, they may also allow favor survival melanoma and squamous cell carcinoma.

Website: http://commons.cit.nih.gov/crisp3/CRISP.Generate_Ticket

- **Project Title:** Development of Mechanoreceptors--Role of Neurotrophins

Principal Investigator & Institution: Szeder, Viktor; Cell Biol, Neurobiol/Anatomy; Medical College of Wisconsin 8701 Watertown Plank Rd Milwaukee, Wi 53226

Timing: Fiscal Year 2000; Project Start 5-AUG-2000

Summary: Merkel cells are slowly adapting sensory receptors in the skin that are innervated by Abeta sensory neurons. Virtually nothing is known about the cellular and molecular mechanisms that control development and innervation of Merkel cells. My advisor, Prof. Grim, and his collaborators have shown that Merkel cells are derived from the neural crest and that their precursors migrate in the ventrolateral migratory pathway in the subectodermal space. The proposed work is designed to elucidate some of the roles growth factors play in the development of quail neural crest cells into Merkel cells. In Aim 1, Merkel cells in culture will be characterized at the ultrastructural level and compared to Merkel cells in the intact organism. In Aim 2, the expression during embryonic development of pertinent growth factor receptors by Merkel cell precursors and maturing Merkel cells will be elucidated by indirect immunohistochemistry and in situ hybridization. Additionally, the autocrine and/or paracrine expression of the receptor ligands will be determined. Candidate growth factors include stem cell factor (SCF), epidermal growth factor (EGF), nerve growth factor (NGF) and neurotrophin-3 (NT-3). By use of the neural crest cell colony assay that has been developed in Prof. Sieber-Blum's laboratory, I propose in Aim 3 to assess the role of pertinent growth factors (as determined in Aim 2) in the survival, proliferation and differentiation of Merkel cells. The proposed work has relevance to human neurological disease. In individuals with anhidrotic ectodermal dysplasia, and in the corresponding mouse model, Tabby, there are no Merkel cells (Srivastava et al., 1997; Vielkind et al., 1995). This is most likely due to down-regulation of the EGF receptor. In vitiligo, Merkel cells as well as melanocytes are lost (Kumar Bose, 1994). A disrupted neurotrophin-3 gene in mice causes perinatal loss of Merkel cells and other neurodegenerative symptoms (Airaksinen et al., 1996). Merkel cell carcinoma (small, intermediate and trabecular types) is a relatively frequent tumor (Schmidt et al., 1998). Insights into the mechanisms that regulate normal Merkel cell development may prove useful in future approaches for the prevention or treatment of neurological disease.

Website: http://commons.cit.nih.gov/crisp3/CRISP.Generate_Ticket

- **Project Title: Molecular Mechanisms of SOD/GSH Genes in Melanocytes**

Principal Investigator & Institution: Bowers, Roger R.; Professor; California State University Los Angeles 5151 State University Dr Los Angeles, Ca 90032

Timing: Fiscal Year 2000; Project Start 4-JUN-1978; Project End 0-JUN-2004

Summary: A hypothesis is proposed for premature death in Barred Plymouth Rock (PBR) and White Leghorn (WL) chicken melanocytes. BPR melanocytes are genetically sensitive due to a defect in their SOD and GSH levels caused by the barring gene and die prematurely from oxygen radical toxicity. WL chickens carry the dominant white gene in addition to the barring gene and have a further reduction of SOD and their melanocytes die much earlier than the BPR melanocytes. Some forms of human vitiligo may be caused by a similar mechanism. The specific aims are focused to further test this hypothesis and to elucidate at the molecular gene level why SOD and GSH levels are low in the mutant birds and to determine the role that the keratinocytes may play in these vitiliginous avian models. The in vivo experiments are as follows: (1) Isolation of Cytosolic (CT) Cu/Zn bird using a competitive reference standard and RT-PCR. Sequence and compare the CT Cu/Zn SOD of the WLH with the BPR and JF. Comparisons will also include other species. Compare and assess differences in CT SOD between the 3 bird types by expression of the enzyme under a single promoter. (2) Analysis of three CT SOD between the 3 bird types by expression of the enzyme under a single promoter. (2) Analysis of three important enzymes in glutathione metabolism will be performed in JF, BPR and WL feature tissue with the JF serving as a control. If the down regulation of GSH is determined to be caused by one or more of the enzymes involved, then a molecular characterization of the mutant gene will be performed in the same manner as that for the SOD gene. (3) A thorough light and electron microscope study of the JF, BPR and WL feature melanocytes and keratinocytes will be performed to determine if any structural aberrations like those described in human vitiligo melanocytes occur in these mutant line cells. Enzymes associated with melanogenesis and cell death will be analyzed cytochemically in the melanocytes. In all cases, the JF will serve as a control. The in vitro studies consist of: (1) establishing the primary melanocyte cultures of the JF, BPR MSH to the media or by not changing the media. (2) Thorough electron microscope studies will be done on these three genotypes of melanocytes in normal and premature death conditions to see if the morphology is similar to that of the in vivo normal and dying melanocytes. (3) Since keratinocytes may play a large role in the survival and differentiation of the melanocytes, SOD, GSH, catalase,. GSH-peroxidase under normal and oxygen radical stress conditions. The measurements of the above parameters of the feather tissue, which predominately includes the keratinocytes and few melanocytes, has already been performed.

Website: http://commons.cit.nih.gov/crisp3/CRISP.Generate_Ticket

- **Project Title: Novel Oligopeptides as Topical Skin Lightening Agents**

Principal Investigator & Institution: Leyda, James P.; Emerging Concepts 3130 Highland Ave, Ste 3115 Cincinnati, Oh 45219

Timing: Fiscal Year 2001; Project Start 1-JUL-2001; Project End 0-JUN-2002

Summary: (Verbatim) - Hyperpigmentary skin disorders affect several millions of people worldwide and are often the cause of social, life style and emotional problems. These disorders include solar lentigines (liver spots), vitiligo, freckles, and darkening of grafted skin. Additionally, the desire for skin whitening cosmetics is common in various cultures around the world. Current treatments lightening skin are usually topically applied harsh chemicals, such as hydroquinone or its derivatives, but overall lack reliability in efficacy and have issues of safety. We have isolated and characterized a unique and potent skin lightening protein from hyperpigmented xenographs. This natural agent provides a new approach to blocking the formation of melanin, the cause of hyperpigmentation. In both in vitro and in vivo models, the protein effectively inhibits the activity of tyrosinase, a marker for hyperpigmentation. A small fragment of the protein has been identified that effectively mimics the in vitro activity. The goals of these Phase I studies are to demonstrate in vivo effectiveness of the fragment and to identify a small series of peptides for optimization and clinical evaluation in Phase II. The effective topical products from Phase II will provide the prototype product for commercialization in Phase III. PROPOSED COMMERCIAL APPLICATION: A topical skin lightening product has significant commercial medical opportunities in the prevention and treatment of skin discoloration disorders and in cosmeceutical use. Burn victims, the aging and other individuals with skin hyperpigmentation exist by the millions throughout the world. This would be a significant market. The cosmeceutical uses expand the potential many fold.

Website: http://commons.cit.nih.gov/crisp3/CRISP.Generate_Ticket

- **Project Title: Preclinical Study of Peptide Based Human Tumor Vaccines**

Principal Investigator & Institution: Engelhard, Victor H.; Associate Professor; Beirne Carter Ctr/Immuno Res; University of Virginia Charlottesville Box 400195 Charlottesville, Va 22904

Timing: Fiscal Year 2000; Project Start 1-SEP-1998; Project End 0-JUN-2003

Summary: (Adapted from the Investigator's Abstract): Peptide antigens presented by class I MHC molecules and recognized by cytotoxic T lymphocytes (CTL) have been defined for several infectious agents and tumors of both murine and human origin. These peptides represent attractive candidates for the development of therapeutic and/or prophylactic vaccines for diseases in which CTL play an important role, including cancer. The technology for appropriate delivery of peptide antigens is still new and undergoing rapid development, and no consensus methodology exists. In addition, while CTL responses against pathogens and tumors have been stimulated by many of these methods, there have also been numerous failures. One important factor in the use of peptide antigens is that their affinity for the presenting MHC molecule will influence the level at which they are presented by APC in order to stimulate a CTL response, as well as their display on an infected cell or a tumor. In this regard, a large set of peptide antigens that are the subject of a number of clinical trials are those that have been defined as CTL targets on human melanoma cells. However, most of these peptides have a relatively low affinity for the presenting molecule HLA-A*0201, and it is not clear how to deliver these antigens in order to stimulate the most effective CTL. In addition, reproducible and generally accepted criteria for the development of effective CTL in response to vaccination are not well established. Therefore, it is important to develop means of quantifying CTL activity that bear a direct relationship to therapeutic efficacy. Comprehensive evaluation of these issues in vaccine delivery methodology in early stage clinical trials is prohibitive because of the difficulty in enrolling significant numbers of patients in many different protocols and comparing results obtained by the use of different methods. Therefore, development of appropriate preclinical models is a desirable goal. The specific aims of this proposal will lead to the definition of methodology to measure both CTL number and avidity, and the use of this methodology to evaluate the importance of these parameters in effective tumor-specific immune responses. In addition, the impact of peptide affinity for MHC molecules on both the stimulation of CTL and their effectiveness in tumor destruction will be examined systematically. These issues will be addressed through the development of a preclinical model that will allow the evaluation of effective immune responses to peptide antigens that are presented by human class I MHC molecules.

Website: http://commons.cit.nih.gov/crisp3/CRISP.Generate_Ticket

E-Journals: PubMed Central[17]

PubMed Central (PMC) is a digital archive of life sciences journal literature developed and managed by the National Center for Biotechnology Information (NCBI) at the U.S. National Library of Medicine (NLM).[18] Access to this growing archive of e-journals is free and unrestricted.[19] To search, go to **http://www.pubmedcentral.nih.gov/index.html#search**, and type "vitiligo" (or synonyms) into the search box. This search gives you access to full-text articles. The following is a sample of items found for vitiligo in the PubMed Central database:

- **Vaccination with a recombinant vaccinia virus encoding a "self" antigen induces autoimmune vitiligo and tumor cell destruction in mice: Requirement for CD4 + T lymphocytes** by Willem W. Overwijk, David S. Lee, Deborah R. Surman, Kari R. Irvine, Christopher E. Touloukian, Chi-Chao Chan, Miles W. Carroll, Bernard Moss, Steven A. Rosenberg, and Nicholas P. Restifo; 1999 March 16
  http://www.pubmedcentral.nih.gov/articlerender.fcgi?artid=15881

The National Library of Medicine: PubMed

One of the quickest and most comprehensive ways to find academic studies in both English and other languages is to use PubMed, maintained by the National Library of Medicine. The advantage of PubMed over previously mentioned sources is that it covers a greater number of domestic and foreign

---

[17] Adapted from the National Library of Medicine:
http://www.pubmedcentral.nih.gov/about/intro.html.
[18] With PubMed Central, NCBI is taking the lead in preservation and maintenance of open access to electronic literature, just as NLM has done for decades with printed biomedical literature. PubMed Central aims to become a world-class library of the digital age.
[19] The value of PubMed Central, in addition to its role as an archive, lies the availability of data from diverse sources stored in a common format in a single repository. Many journals already have online publishing operations, and there is a growing tendency to publish material online only, to the exclusion of print.

references. It is also free to the public.[20] If the publisher has a Web site that offers full text of its journals, PubMed will provide links to that site, as well as to sites offering other related data. User registration, a subscription fee, or some other type of fee may be required to access the full text of articles in some journals.

To generate your own bibliography of studies dealing with vitiligo, simply go to the PubMed Web site at **www.ncbi.nlm.nih.gov/pubmed**. Type "vitiligo" (or synonyms) into the search box, and click "Go." The following is the type of output you can expect from PubMed for "vitiligo" (hyperlinks lead to article summaries):

- **Childhood vitiligo successfully treated with bath PUVA.**
  Author(s): Mai DW, Omohundro C, Dijkstra JW, Bailin PL.
  Source: Pediatr Dermatol. 1998 January-February; 15(1): 53-5.
  http://www.ncbi.nlm.nih.gov:80/entrez/query.fcgi?cmd=Retrieve&db=PubMed&list_uids=9496807&dopt=Abstract

- **Improvement of vitiligo after oral treatment with vitamin B12 and folic acid and the importance of sun exposure.**
  Author(s): Juhlin L, Olsson MJ.
  Source: Acta Derm Venereol. 1997 November; 77(6): 460-2.
  http://www.ncbi.nlm.nih.gov:80/entrez/query.fcgi?cmd=Retrieve&db=PubMed&list_uids=9394983&dopt=Abstract

- **Vitiligo--a retrospect.**
  Author(s): Nair BK.
  Source: Int J Dermatol. 1978 November; 17(9): 755-7. No Abstract Available.
  http://www.ncbi.nlm.nih.gov:80/entrez/query.fcgi?cmd=Retrieve&db=PubMed&list_uids=365814&dopt=Abstract

Vocabulary Builder

Aberrant: Wandering or deviating from the usual or normal course. [EU]

---

[20] PubMed was developed by the National Center for Biotechnology Information (NCBI) at the National Library of Medicine (NLM) at the National Institutes of Health (NIH). The PubMed database was developed in conjunction with publishers of biomedical literature as a search tool for accessing literature citations and linking to full-text journal articles at Web sites of participating publishers. Publishers that participate in PubMed supply NLM with their citations electronically prior to or at the time of publication.

Acrodermatitis: Inflammation involving the skin of the extremities, especially the hands and feet. Several forms are known, some idiopathic and some hereditary. The infantile form is called Gianotti-Crosti syndrome. [NIH]

Alleles: Mutually exclusive forms of the same gene, occupying the same locus on homologous chromosomes, and governing the same biochemical and developmental process. [NIH]

Allylamine: Possesses an unusual and selective cytotoxicity for vascular smooth muscle cells in dogs and rats. Useful for experiments dealing with arterial injury, myocardial fibrosis or cardiac decompensation. [NIH]

Analogous: Resembling or similar in some respects, as in function or appearance, but not in origin or development;. [EU]

Antigen: Any substance which is capable, under appropriate conditions, of inducing a specific immune response and of reacting with the products of that response, that is, with specific antibody or specifically sensitized T-lymphocytes, or both. Antigens may be soluble substances, such as toxins and foreign proteins, or particulate, such as bacteria and tissue cells; however, only the portion of the protein or polysaccharide molecule known as the antigenic determinant (q.v.) combines with antibody or a specific receptor on a lymphocyte. Abbreviated Ag. [EU]

Antioxidant: One of many widely used synthetic or natural substances added to a product to prevent or delay its deterioration by action of oxygen in the air. Rubber, paints, vegetable oils, and prepared foods commonly contain antioxidants. [EU]

Arginine: An essential amino acid that is physiologically active in the L-form. [NIH]

Assay: Determination of the amount of a particular constituent of a mixture, or of the biological or pharmacological potency of a drug. [EU]

Atopic: Pertaining to an atopen or to atopy; allergic. [EU]

Auditory: Pertaining to the sense of hearing. [EU]

Biochemical: Relating to biochemistry; characterized by, produced by, or involving chemical reactions in living organisms. [EU]

Bullous: Pertaining to or characterized by bullae. [EU]

Candidiasis: Infection with a fungus of the genus Candida. It is usually a superficial infection of the moist cutaneous areas of the body, and is generally caused by C. albicans; it most commonly involves the skin (dermatocandidiasis), oral mucous membranes (thrush, def. 1), respiratory tract (bronchocandidiasis), and vagina (vaginitis). Rarely there is a systemic infection or endocarditis. Called also moniliasis, candidosis, oidiomycosis, and formerly blastodendriosis. [EU]

Carcinoma: A malignant new growth made up of epithelial cells tending to infiltrate the surrounding tissues and give rise to metastases. [EU]

Catalase: An oxidoreductase that catalyzes the conversion of hydrogen peroxide to water and oxygen. It is present in many animal cells. A deficiency of this enzyme results in ACATALASIA. EC 1.11.1.6. [NIH]

Catechols: A group of 1,2-benzenediols that contain the general formula R-C6H5O2. [NIH]

Clotrimazole: An imidazole derivative with a broad spectrum of antimycotic activity. It inhibits biosynthesis of the sterol ergostol, an important component of fungal cell membranes. Its action leads to increased membrane permeability and apparent disruption of enzyme systems bound to the membrane. [NIH]

Cutaneous: Pertaining to the skin; dermal; dermic. [EU]

Cytokines: Non-antibody proteins secreted by inflammatory leukocytes and some non-leukocytic cells, that act as intercellular mediators. They differ from classical hormones in that they are produced by a number of tissue or cell types rather than by specialized glands. They generally act locally in a paracrine or autocrine rather than endocrine manner. [NIH]

Cytomegalovirus: A genus of the family herpesviridae, subfamily betaherpesvirinae, infecting the salivary glands, liver, spleen, lungs, eyes, and other organs, in which they produce characteristically enlarged cells with intranuclear inclusions. Infection with Cytomegalovirus is also seen as an opportunistic infection in AIDS. [NIH]

Dermatophytosis: Any superficial fungal infection caused by a dermatophyte and involving the stratum corneum of the skin, hair, and nails. The term broadly comprises onychophytosis and the various form of tinea (ringworm), sometimes being used specifically to designate tinea pedis (athlete's foot). Called also epidermomycosis. [EU]

Dysplasia: Abnormality of development; in pathology, alteration in size, shape, and organization of adult cells. [EU]

Econazole: A broad spectrum antimycotic with some action against Gram positive bacteria. It is used topically in dermatomycoses also orally and parenterally. [NIH]

Eczema: A pruritic papulovesicular dermatitis occurring as a reaction to many endogenous and exogenous agents, characterized in the acute stage by erythema, edema associated with a serous exudate between the cells of the epidermis (spongiosis) and an inflammatory infiltrate in the dermis, oozing and vesiculation, and crusting and scaling; and in the more chronic stages by lichenification or thickening or both, signs of excoriations, and hyperpigmentation or hypopigmentation or both. Atopic dermatitis is the most common type of dermatitis. Called also eczematous dermatitis. [EU]

Enzyme: A protein molecule that catalyses chemical reactions of other substances without itself being destroyed or altered upon completion of the reactions. Enzymes are classified according to the recommendations of the Nomenclature Committee of the International Union of Biochemistry. Each enzyme is assigned a recommended name and an Enzyme Commission (EC) number. They are divided into six main groups; oxidoreductases, transferases, hydrolases, lyases, isomerases, and ligases. [EU]

Epidemiological: Relating to, or involving epidemiology. [EU]

Epidermal: Pertaining to or resembling epidermis. Called also epidermic or epidermoid. [EU]

Erythrasma: A chronic, superficial bacterial infection of the skin involving the body folds and toe webs, sometimes becoming generalized, caused by Corynebacterium minutissimum, and characterized by the presence of sharply demarcated, dry, brown, slightly scaly, and slowly spreading patches. [EU]

Fissure: Any cleft or groove, normal or otherwise; especially a deep fold in the cerebral cortex which involves the entire thickness of the brain wall. [EU]

Fistula: An abnormal passage or communication, usually between two internal organs, or leading from an internal organ to the surface of the body; frequently designated according to the organs or parts with which it communicates, as anovaginal, brochocutaneous, hepatopleural, pulmonoperitoneal, rectovaginal, urethrovaginal, and the like. Such passages are frequently created experimentally for the purpose of obtaining body secretions for physiologic study. [EU]

Fluconazole: Triazole antifungal agent that is used to treat oropharyngeal candidiasis and cryptococcal meningitis in AIDS. [NIH]

Genotype: The genetic constitution of the individual; the characterization of the genes. [NIH]

Griseofulvin: An antifungal antibiotic. Griseofulvin may be given by mouth in the treatment of tinea infections. [NIH]

Homeostasis: A tendency to stability in the normal body states (internal environment) of the organism. It is achieved by a system of control mechanisms activated by negative feedback; e.g. a high level of carbon dioxide in extracellular fluid triggers increased pulmonary ventilation, which in turn causes a decrease in carbon dioxide concentration. [EU]

Humoral: Of, relating to, proceeding from, or involving a bodily humour - now often used of endocrine factors as opposed to neural or somatic. [EU]

Hybridization: The genetic process of crossbreeding to produce a hybrid. Hybrid nucleic acids can be formed by nucleic acid hybridization of DNA and RNA molecules. Protein hybridization allows for hybrid proteins to be formed from polypeptide chains. [NIH]

Hydrogen: Hydrogen. The first chemical element in the periodic table. It has the atomic symbol H, atomic number 1, and atomic weight 1. It exists, under normal conditions, as a colorless, odorless, tasteless, diatomic gas. Hydrogen ions are protons. Besides the common H1 isotope, hydrogen exists as the stable isotope deuterium and the unstable, radioactive isotope tritium. [NIH]

Immunohistochemistry: Histochemical localization of immunoreactive substances using labeled antibodies as reagents. [NIH]

Incubation: The development of an infectious disease from the entrance of the pathogen to the appearance of clinical symptoms. [EU]

Induction: The act or process of inducing or causing to occur, especially the production of a specific morphogenetic effect in the developing embryo through the influence of evocators or organizers, or the production of anaesthesia or unconsciousness by use of appropriate agents. [EU]

Innervation: 1. the distribution or supply of nerves to a part. 2. the supply of nervous energy or of nerve stimulus sent to a part. [EU]

Insulin: A protein hormone secreted by beta cells of the pancreas. Insulin plays a major role in the regulation of glucose metabolism, generally promoting the cellular utilization of glucose. It is also an important regulator of protein and lipid metabolism. Insulin is used as a drug to control insulin-dependent diabetes mellitus. [NIH]

Intertrigo: A superficial dermatitis occurring on apposed skin surfaces, such as the axillae, creases of the neck, intergluteal fold, groin, between the toes, and beneath pendulous breasts, with obesity being a predisposing factor, caused by moisture, friction, warmth, and sweat retention, and characterized by erythema, maceration, burning, itching, and sometimes erosions, fissures, and exudations and secondary infections. Called also eczema intertrigo. [EU]

Itraconazole: An antifungal agent that has been used in the treatment of histoplasmosis, blastomycosis, cryptococcal meningitis, and aspergillosis. [NIH]

Ketoconazole: Broad spectrum antifungal agent used for long periods at high doses, especially in immunosuppressed patients. [NIH]

Leprosy: A chronic granulomatous infection caused by mycobacterium LEPRAE. The granulomatous lesions are manifested in the skin, the mucous membranes, and the peripheral nerves. Two polar or principal types are lepromatous and tuberculoid. [NIH]

Maceration: The softening of a solid by soaking. In histology, the softening of a tissue by soaking, especially in acids, until the connective tissue fibres are so dissolved that the tissue components can be teased apart. In obstetrics, the degenerative changes with discoloration and softening of tissues, and eventual disintegration, of a fetus retained in the uterus after its death. [EU]

Mechanoreceptors: Cells specialized to transduce mechanical stimuli and relay that information centrally in the nervous system. Mechanoreceptors include hair cells, which mediate hearing and balance, and the various somatosensory receptors, often with non-neural accessory structures. [NIH]

Mediator: An object or substance by which something is mediated, such as (1) a structure of the nervous system that transmits impulses eliciting a specific response; (2) a chemical substance (transmitter substance) that induces activity in an excitable tissue, such as nerve or muscle; or (3) a substance released from cells as the result of the interaction of antigen with antibody or by the action of antigen with a sensitized lymphocyte. [EU]

Melanosomes: Melanin-containing organelles found in melanocytes and melanophores. [NIH]

Miconazole: An imidazole antifungal agent that is used topically and by intravenous infusion. [NIH]

Molecular: Of, pertaining to, or composed of molecules : a very small mass of matter. [EU]

Mucosa: A mucous membrane, or tunica mucosa. [EU]

Necrolysis: Separation or exfoliation of tissue due to necrosis. [EU]

Neural: 1. pertaining to a nerve or to the nerves. 2. situated in the region of the spinal axis, as the neutral arch. [EU]

Neurons: The basic cellular units of nervous tissue. Each neuron consists of a body, an axon, and dendrites. Their purpose is to receive, conduct, and transmit impulses in the nervous system. [NIH]

Nystatin: Macrolide antifungal antibiotic complex produced by Streptomyces noursei, S. aureus, and other Streptomyces species. The biologically active components of the complex are nystatin A1, A2, and A3. [NIH]

Ocular: 1. of, pertaining to, or affecting the eye. 2. eyepiece. [EU]

Oligopeptides: Peptides composed of between two and twelve amino acids. [NIH]

Perinatal: Pertaining to or occurring in the period shortly before and after birth; variously defined as beginning with completion of the twentieth to twenty-eighth week of gestation and ending 7 to 28 days after birth. [EU]

Peroxidase: A hemeprotein from leukocytes. Deficiency of this enzyme leads to a hereditary disorder coupled with disseminated moniliasis. It catalyzes the conversion of a donor and peroxide to an oxidized donor and water. EC 1.11.1.7. [NIH]

Phenotype: The outward appearance of the individual. It is the product of interactions between genes and between the genotype and the environment. This includes the killer phenotype, characteristic of yeasts. [NIH]

Polymorphic: Occurring in several or many forms; appearing in different forms at different stages of development. [EU]

Postnatal: Occurring after birth, with reference to the newborn. [EU]

Preclinical: Before a disease becomes clinically recognizable. [EU]

Precursor: Something that precedes. In biological processes, a substance from which another, usually more active or mature substance is formed. In clinical medicine, a sign or symptom that heralds another. [EU]

Proximal: Nearest; closer to any point of reference; opposed to distal. [EU]

Pustular: Pertaining to or of the nature of a pustule; consisting of pustules (= a visible collection of pus within or beneath the epidermis). [EU]

Pyoderma: Any purulent skin disease. Called also pyodermia. [EU]

Receptor: 1. a molecular structure within a cell or on the surface characterized by (1) selective binding of a specific substance and (2) a specific physiologic effect that accompanies the binding, e.g., cell-surface receptors for peptide hormones, neurotransmitters, antigens, complement fragments, and immunoglobulins and cytoplasmic receptors for steroid hormones. 2. a sensory nerve terminal that responds to stimuli of various kinds. [EU]

Recombinant: 1. a cell or an individual with a new combination of genes not found together in either parent; usually applied to linked genes. [EU]

Sarcoma: A tumour made up of a substance like the embryonic connective tissue; tissue composed of closely packed cells embedded in a fibrillar or homogeneous substance. Sarcomas are often highly malignant. [EU]

Selenium: An element with the atomic symbol Se, atomic number 34, and atomic weight 78.96. It is an essential micronutrient for mammals and other animals but is toxic in large amounts. Selenium protects intracellular structures against oxidative damage. It is an essential component of glutathione peroxidase. [NIH]

Serum: The clear portion of any body fluid; the clear fluid moistening serous membranes. 2. blood serum; the clear liquid that separates from blood on clotting. 3. immune serum; blood serum from an immunized animal used for passive immunization; an antiserum; antitoxin, or antivenin. [EU]

Toxin: A poison; frequently used to refer specifically to a protein produced by some higher plants, certain animals, and pathogenic bacteria, which is highly toxic for other living organisms. Such substances are differentiated from the simple chemical poisons and the vegetable alkaloids by their high molecular weight and antigenicity. [EU]

Ulceration: 1. the formation or development of an ulcer. 2. an ulcer. [EU]

Vaccination: The introduction of vaccine into the body for the purpose of inducing immunity. Coined originally to apply to the injection of smallpox vaccine, the term has come to mean any immunizing procedure in which vaccine is injected. [EU]

Vaccine: A suspension of attenuated or killed microorganisms (bacteria, viruses, or rickettsiae), administered for the prevention, amelioration or treatment of infectious diseases. [EU]

Varicella: Chicken pox. [EU]

Vasculitis: Inflammation of a vessel, angiitis. [EU]

Warts: Benign epidermal proliferations or tumors; some are viral in origin. [NIH]

CHAPTER 4. PATENTS ON VITILIGO

Overview

You can learn about innovations relating to vitiligo by reading recent patents and patent applications. Patents can be physical innovations (e.g. chemicals, pharmaceuticals, medical equipment) or processes (e.g. treatments or diagnostic procedures). The United States Patent and Trademark Office defines a patent as a grant of a property right to the inventor, issued by the Patent and Trademark Office.[21] Patents, therefore, are intellectual property. For the United States, the term of a new patent is 20 years from the date when the patent application was filed. If the inventor wishes to receive economic benefits, it is likely that the invention will become commercially available to patients with vitiligo within 20 years of the initial filing. It is important to understand, therefore, that an inventor's patent does not indicate that a product or service is or will be commercially available to patients with vitiligo. The patent implies only that the inventor has "the right to exclude others from making, using, offering for sale, or selling" the invention in the United States. While this relates to U.S. patents, similar rules govern foreign patents.

In this chapter, we show you how to locate information on patents and their inventors. If you find a patent that is particularly interesting to you, contact the inventor or the assignee for further information.

---

[21]Adapted from The U. S. Patent and Trademark Office: **http://www.uspto.gov/web/offices/pac/doc/general/whatis.htm**.

Patents on Vitiligo

By performing a patent search focusing on vitiligo, you can obtain information such as the title of the invention, the names of the inventor(s), the assignee(s) or the company that owns or controls the patent, a short abstract that summarizes the patent, and a few excerpts from the description of the patent. The abstract of a patent tends to be more technical in nature, while the description is often written for the public. Full patent descriptions contain much more information than is presented here (e.g. claims, references, figures, diagrams, etc.). We will tell you how to obtain this information later in the chapter. The following is an example of the type of information that you can expect to obtain from a patent search on vitiligo:

- **Process for the preparation of an extract from human placenta containing glycosphingolipids and endothelin-like constituent peptides useful for the treatment of vitiligo**

  Inventor(s): Bhadra; Ranjan (Calcutta, IN), Pal; Prajnamoy (Calcutta, IN), Roy; Rabindra (Dickinson, TX), Dutta; Ajit Kumar (Calcutta, IN)

  Assignee(s): Council of Scientific & Industrial Research (IN)

  Patent Number: 5,690,966

  Date filed: October 17, 1996

  Abstract: A process for the preparation of an extract from human placenta containing glycosphingolipids and endothelin-like peptides useful for the treatment of vitiligo is disclosed.

  Excerpt(s): Vitiligo or `Swetakustha`, as described in ancient medical text, is a skin disfiguring phenomenon affecting about 1% of the world population compared to 3% Indians. Though not painful or lethal in nature but patients burdened with mental agony and depression due to social stigma, are extremely eager to have a wholly satisfactory-therapy for this disease. Unfortunately, vitiligo failed to respond in many oases with the therapies currently in use. So to develop a therapy satisfying the desired parameters has remained as a challenge to modern medical science. ... Among the therapies mostly ill-defined, human placental extract has been claimed to be effective for vitiligo without proper justification by scientific investigation namely indication of the active components. Still the method of preparation of the extract is secretly guarded. ... Regarding the efficacy of the available placental extract used in the treatment of vitiligo a lot of criticisms have been cropped up from different scientific quarters (Nordlund J. J., Halder R. Melagenina--An analysis of published and other available data. Dermatologica 1990; 181: 1-4; Goldstein E., Haberman H. F., Menon I. A., Pawlowski D. Non-psoralen treatment of vitiligo. Part II. Less commonly used and Experimental Therapies. Int. J. Dermatol. 1992; 31: 314-319) primarily for the lack of scientific evidences in respect of active principles present in it. But all the critics instead of discarding it as therapy, stressed the need for a thorough and intensive scientific investigation to look for the active components of the extracts. Some recent reports (Kojima N., Hakomori Sen-itiroth--Cell adhesion, spreading and motility of GM3-expressing cells based on glycolipid-glycolipid interaction. J. Biol. Chem. 1991; 266: 17552-17558; Imokawa G., Yada Y., Miyagishi M. Endothelin secreted from human kerationcytes are intrinsic mitogens for human melanocytes. J. Biol. Chem. 1992; 267: 24675-24680) in this respect described that glycosphingolipids and a 21-amino acid vasocons-trictor peptide, endothelin are the potent modulators of melanocyte migration as well as motility and growth promotion respectively. These are the key events in the recovery of skin pigmentation.

Web site: http://www.delphion.com/details?pn=US05690966__

- **Method and composition for treating vitiligo**

  Inventor(s): Montes; Leopoldo F. (Buenos Aires, AR)

  Assignee(s): none reported

  Patent Number: 4,985,443

  Date filed: August 4, 1989

  Abstract: To cure vitiligo without side effects, a disease characterized by cutaneous depigmentation, a treatment consisting in the oral administration of folic acid in daily doses from 1 to 50 mg. The treatment of vitiligo with folic acid can be enhanced by also using oral vitamin C and intramuscular vitamin B.sub.12.

  Excerpt(s): The present invention deals with a new treatment of patients having vitiligo be means of chemical compositions containing folic acid. ... Vitiligo is a disease which affects 1%-2% of the world population according to J. A Rook, D. S. Wilkinson and F. J. G. Ebling (Textbook to Dermatology, Blackwell Scientific Publications, Oxford, 1979). ... It results from the lack of melanin in the epidrmis due to the disappearance of melanocytes from the epidermis, as it is defined by A. S. Breathnach, S. Bohr and L. M. Wyllie in "Electron Microscopy of Peripheral Nerve Terminals and Marginal Melanocytes in Vitiligo", J. Invest. Dermat. 47:125-140, 1966.

  Web site: http://www.delphion.com/details?pn=US04985443__

Patent Applications on Vitiligo

As of December 2000, U.S. patent applications are open to public viewing.[22] Applications are patent requests which have yet to be granted (the process to achieve a patent can take several years). The following patent applications have been filed since December 2000 relating to vitiligo:

- **Treatment of vitiligo**

    Inventor(s): Spencer, James M. ; (New York, NY)

    Correspondence: DARBY & DARBY P.C.; 805 Third Avenue; New York; NY; 10022-7513; US

    Patent Application Number: 20020013609

    Date filed: February 22, 2001

    Abstract: Disclosed herein is a novel method of treating vitiligo by using an excimer laser that emits light in the UVB range. The invention includes a method of incrementally increasing exposure of affected vitiligo areas with UVB laser light from an excimer laser to restore pigmentation to skin areas afflicted with vitiligo.

    Excerpt(s): Vitiligo is a cutaneous disease in which there is a complete loss of pigment in localized areas of the skin. This loss of pigment results in the effected areas being completely white. This condition has a predilection for the skin around the mouth and the eyes. The result is cosmetically disfiguring, especially for dark skinned people. Furthermore, the depigmented skin is sun sensitive, and thus is subject to sunburns and skin cancer. In sum, vitiligo is both cosmetically and practically distressing to patients afflicted with the disease. ... In normal skin, varying shades of brown are seen (depending on a person's race) representing the pigment melanin. This pigment is produced by a cell type known as a melanocyte. In vitiligo, there is an absence of melanocytes in the areas afflicted with the disorder. An absence of melanocytes results in an absence of melanin pigment, and thus the melanin-free area is white. Normal skin responds to ultraviolet light with an increase in the brown pigment melanin (tanning). Specifically, ultraviolet radiation stimulates melanocytes to proliferate and produce more melanin. ... Attempts have also been made to "tan" vitiligo areas using ultraviolet light treatments. The ultraviolet spectrum is divided into two portions, "UVA" and "UVB," which is light of 320-400 nm and 290-320 nm in wavelength, respectively. UVB is much more effective at producing a tan in normal skin. In normal skin, melanocytes reside in the

---

[22] This has been a common practice outside the United States prior to December 2000.

epidermis, which is the outer layer of the skin. The epidermis is only 0.1 mm thick, so the melanocytes are very near the surface. UVB radiation can only penetrate to about 0.1 mm, but this is sufficient to reach the melanocytes. In patients with vitiligo, these epidermal melanocytes are gone. In some cases, there are surviving melanocytes deeper in the skin down the hair follicles. These melanocytes may be several millimeters deep. UVB cannot penetrate this deep in the skin to stimulate these surviving deep melanocytes. Exposure to UVB results in a sunburn at the surface of the skin with no stimulation of these deep melanocytes. Thus attempts to repopulate the vitiligo areas with melanocytes deep in the skin in response to UVB exposure have failed. UVA will penetrate a bit deeper in the skin than UVB. However, UVA is very poor at stimulating melanocytes to proliferate and migrate.

Web site: http://appft1.uspto.gov/netahtml/PTO/search-bool.html

- **Composition and method for the treatment of vitiligo**

Inventor(s): Zhao, Huiping ; (Etobicoke, CA)

Correspondence: Gifford, Krass, Groh, Sprinkle; Anderson & Citkowski, PC; 280 N Old Woodard Ave; Suite 400; birmingham; MI; 48009; US

Patent Application Number: 20010044422

Date filed: December 28, 2000

Abstract: Compositions and methods for the treatment of vitiligo. The composition comprises at least one member selected from the group consisting of: Eclipta prostrata L., Angelica dahurica (Fish. ex. Hoffm), Polygonum multiforum Thumb, Astragalus complanatus, Tribulus terrestris L., Lithospermum erythrorhizon sieb et zucc, Paris petiolata (Bak. ex Forb), Salvia multiorrhiza Bge, Sophora flavescens Ait, Atractylodes lancea (Thumb) Dc, and combinations thereof. The method comprises treating the vitiligo by orally administering this composition to the patient. The treatment may be further enhanced by topically administering to the affected areas a composition selected from the group consisting of: a preparation of sulfur and kerosene; a preparation of Nevlum oporum solund and alcohol; a preparation of Cinnamomum cassia presl, Psoralea corylifalia L., alcohol and water; and a preparation of Portulaca oleracea L., brown sugar, and vinegar.

Excerpt(s): This invention relates generally to treatment of skin conditions and, more specifically, to the treatment of vitiligo. Most specifically, the invention relates to compositions for the treatment of vitiligo, and methods for their use. ... Vitiligo, also referred to as leucoderma, is a skin condition characterized by patchy loss of pigmentation from a person's skin. The specific causes of vitiligo are unknown; however, the depigmented areas are lacking in the skin pigment melanin, and it is believed that the disease is the result of the destruction or inhibition of the melanin secreting melanocytes in the affected areas. There may be some hereditary component to the disease, since approximately 30% of the cases have a familial correlation. It is speculated that the disease may be the result of an autoimmune condition. It is also possible that a specific metabolic defect may be involved, and in some instances, environmental factors appear to play a role. ... In some instances, vitiligo can be treated with topical corticosteroids, which can stimulate melanin production, possibly by reducing immune reactions. In some instances, melanin production is stimulated by treating the patient with photosensitizing drugs such as psoralen, and then exposing the affected areas of the patient to ultraviolet light. In those instances where the depigmentation is not too extreme, cosmetic preparations may be used as a cover up. Some limited use of skin grafts has also been made. In many instances, treatment is unsuccessful, and some patients opt for chemical bleaching of the remaining pigmented skin so as to produce an even complexion. As will be appreciated, the foregoing treatments are often very harsh and frequently ineffective. Therefore, there is still a need for improved treatment methodologies.

Web site: http://appft1.uspto.gov/netahtml/PTO/search-bool.html

Keeping Current

In order to stay informed about patents and patent applications dealing with vitiligo, you can access the U.S. Patent Office archive via the Internet at no cost to you. This archive is available at the following Web address: **http://www.uspto.gov/main/patents.htm**. Under "Services," click on "Search Patents." You will see two broad options: (1) Patent Grants, and (2) Patent Applications. To see a list of granted patents, perform the following steps: Under "Patent Grants," click "Quick Search." Then, type "vitiligo" (or synonyms) into the "Term 1" box. After clicking on the search button, scroll down to see the various patents which have been granted to date on vitiligo. You can also use this procedure to view pending patent applications concerning vitiligo. Simply go back to the following Web address: **http://www.uspto.gov/main/patents.htm**. Under "Services," click on "Search Patents." Select "Quick Search" under "Patent Applications." Then proceed with the steps listed above.

Vocabulary Builder

Intramuscular: Within the substance of a muscle. [EU]

Kerosene: A refined petroleum fraction used as a fuel as well as a solvent. [NIH]

Microscopy: The application of microscope magnification to the study of materials that cannot be properly seen by the unaided eye. [NIH]

Modulator: A specific inductor that brings out characteristics peculiar to a definite region. [EU]

Motility: The ability to move spontaneously. [EU]

Placenta: A highly vascular fetal organ through which the fetus absorbs oxygen and other nutrients and excretes carbon dioxide and other wastes. It begins to form about the eighth day of gestation when the blastocyst adheres to the decidua. [NIH]

Sulfur: An element that is a member of the chalcogen family. It has an atomic symbol S, atomic number 16, and atomic weight 32.066. It is found in the amino acids cysteine and methionine. [NIH]

CHAPTER 5. BOOKS ON VITILIGO

Overview

This chapter provides bibliographic book references relating to vitiligo. You have many options to locate books on vitiligo. The simplest method is to go to your local bookseller and inquire about titles that they have in stock or can special order for you. Some patients, however, feel uncomfortable approaching their local booksellers and prefer online sources (e.g. **www.amazon.com** and **www.bn.com**). In addition to online booksellers, excellent sources for book titles on vitiligo include the Combined Health Information Database and the National Library of Medicine. Once you have found a title that interests you, visit your local public or medical library to see if it is available for loan.

Book Summaries: Online Booksellers

Commercial Internet-based booksellers, such as Amazon.com and Barnes & Noble.com, offer summaries which have been supplied by each title's publisher. Some summaries also include customer reviews. Your local bookseller may have access to in-house and commercial databases that index all published books (e.g. Books in Print®). The following have been recently listed with online booksellers as relating to vitiligo (sorted alphabetically by title; follow the hyperlink to view more details at Amazon.com):

- **Alopecia and Vitiligo in Autoimmune Polyendocrine Syndrome Type I (Comprehensive Summaries of Uppsala Dissertations, 935)** by Hakan Hedstrand (2000); ISBN: 9155447333;

http://www.amazon.com/exec/obidos/ASIN/9155447333/icongroupin terna

- **Vitiligo & Piebaldism : Treatment of Leucoderma by Transplantation of Autologous Melanocytes (Comprehensive Summaries of Uppsala Dissertations from th** by Mats J. Olsson; ISBN: 9155450806; http://www.amazon.com/exec/obidos/ASIN/9155450806/icongroupin terna

- **Vitiligo : nutritional therapy** by Leopoldo F. Montes; ISBN: 9879624009; http://www.amazon.com/exec/obidos/ASIN/9879624009/icongroupin terna

- **Vitiligo and Other Hypomelanoses of Hair and Skin** by Jean-Paul Ortonne; ISBN: 0306409747; http://www.amazon.com/exec/obidos/ASIN/0306409747/icongroupin terna

- **Vitiligo: A Monograph on the Basic and Clinical Science** by Seung-Kung Hann (Editor), et al; ISBN: 0632050713; http://www.amazon.com/exec/obidos/ASIN/0632050713/icongroupin terna

The National Library of Medicine Book Index

The National Library of Medicine at the National Institutes of Health has a massive database of books published on healthcare and biomedicine. Go to the following Internet site, **http://locatorplus.gov/**, and then select "Search LOCATORplus." Once you are in the search area, simply type "vitiligo" (or synonyms) into the search box, and select "books only." From there, results can be sorted by publication date, author, or relevance. The following was recently catalogued by the National Library of Medicine:[23]

- **Comparative study of albinism, partial albinism, and vitiligo in man with reference to the presence and activity of melanocytes in areas of**

---

[23] In addition to LOCATORPlus, in collaboration with authors and publishers, the National Center for Biotechnology Information (NCBI) is adapting biomedical books for the Web. The books may be accessed in two ways: (1) by searching directly using any search term or phrase (in the same way as the bibliographic database PubMed), or (2) by following the links to PubMed abstracts. Each PubMed abstract has a "Books" button that displays a facsimile of the abstract in which some phrases are hypertext links. These phrases are also found in the books available at NCBI. Click on hyperlinked results in the list of books in which the phrase is found. Currently, the majority of the links are between the books and PubMed. In the future, more links will be created between the books and other types of information, such as gene and protein sequences and macromolecular structures. See **http://www.ncbi.nlm.nih.gov/entrez/query.fcgi?db=Books.**

hypopigmentation; presentation of histological material with a discussion of techniques and review of the literatur.   Author: Kugelman, Thomas Peter; Year: 1960; [New Haven, Dept. of Internal Medicine, Yale Univ. School of Medicine, 1960

- **Genetic, biochemical, and cytochemical studies on leucoderma-vitiligo: report, 1975-1980.**   Author: V.C. Shah; Year: 1982; Ahmedabad: Gujarat University, 1982

- **Immunology of the skin and the eye.**   Author: editors, Manfred Zierhut, Hans-Jürgen Thiel; Year: 1999; Buren, The Netherlands: Aeolus Press, c1999; ISBN: 9070430274
  http://www.amazon.com/exec/obidos/ASIN/9070430274/icongroupin terna

- **Vitiligo: a monograph on the basic and clinical science edited by Seung-kyung Hann and James J. Nordlund; foreword by Aaron B. Lerner.**   Author: Montes, Leopoldo F; Year: 2000; Oxford; Malden, MA: Blackwell Science, 2000; ISBN: 0632050713
  http://www.amazon.com/exec/obidos/ASIN/0632050713/icongroupin terna

- **Vitiligo: neural and immunologic linkages.**   Author: A.K. Dutta; Year: 1988; Calcutta: Indira Publication, 1988

- **Vitiligo: nutritional therapy.**   Author: Leopoldo F. Montes; Year: 1997; [Buenos Aires, Argentina]: Westhoven Press, [c1997]; ISBN: 9879624009
  http://www.amazon.com/exec/obidos/ASIN/9879624009/icongroupin terna

- **Vitiligo and other hypomelanoses of hair and skin.**   Author: Jean Paul Ortonne, David B. Mosher, and Thomas B. Fitzpatrick; Year: 1983; New York: Plenum Medical, c1983; ISBN: 0306409747
  http://www.amazon.com/exec/obidos/ASIN/0306409747/icongroupin terna

- **Vitiligo and psoralens.**   Author: El-Mofty, Abdel Monem; Year: 1968; Oxford, New York, Pergamon [c1968]

Chapters on Vitiligo

Frequently, vitiligo will be discussed within a book, perhaps within a specific chapter. In order to find chapters that are specifically dealing with vitiligo, an excellent source of abstracts is the Combined Health Information Database. You will need to limit your search to book chapters and vitiligo using the "Detailed Search" option. Go directly to the following hyperlink: **http://chid.nih.gov/detail/detail.html**. To find book chapters, use the drop boxes at the bottom of the search page where "You may refine your search by." Select the dates and language you prefer, and the format option "Book Chapter." By making these selections and typing in "vitiligo" (or synonyms) into the "For these words:" box, you will only receive results on chapters in books. The following is a typical result when searching for book chapters on vitiligo:

- **Genetic Hearing Loss Associated with Eye Disorders**

  Source: in Gorlin, R.J.; Toriello, H.V.; Cohen, M.M., Jr., eds. Hereditary Hearing Loss and Its Syndromes. New York, NY: Oxford University Press. 1995. p. 105-140.

  Contact: Available from Oxford University Press. 200 Madison Avenue, New York, NY 10016. (800) 334-4249 or (212) 679-7300. Price: $195.00 plus shipping and handling. ISBN: 0195065522.

  Summary: This chapter, from a text on hereditary hearing loss and its syndromes, discusses genetic hearing loss associated with eye disorders. Conditions covered include Usher syndrome (retinitis pigmentosis and sensorineural hearing loss); Alstrom syndrome; Edwards syndrome; retinitis pigmentosa, nystagmus, hemiplegic migraine, and sensorineural hearing loss; retinitis pigmentosa, vitiligo, and sensorineural hearing loss; Hersh syndrome; choroideremia, obesity, and congenital sensorineural hearing loss; Refsum syndrome; infantile Refsum syndrome; inverse retinitis pigmentosa, hypogonadism, and sensorineural hearing loss; miscellaneous disorders of pigmentary retinopathy and sensorineural hearing loss; myopia and congenital sensorineural hearing loss; Marshall syndrome; Holmes-Schepens syndrome; Harboyan syndrome; familial band keratopathy, abnormal calcium metabolism, and hearing loss; Ehlers-Danlos syndrome, type IV; corneal anesthesia, retinal abnormalities, mental retardation, unusual facies, and sensorineural hearing loss; DeHauwere syndrome; Abruzzo-Erickson syndrome; aniridia and sensorineural hearing loss; congenital total color blindness, cataracts, hyperinsulinism, and sensorineural hearing loss; total color blindness, liver degeneration, endocrine dysfunction, and sensorineural hearing loss; rod-cone dystrophy, renal dysfunction, and sensorineural hearing loss; OHAHA syndrome; IVIC syndrome; cataracts and progressive sensorineural hearing loss; Ohdo syndrome; Michels syndrome; Fraser syndrome; ocular albinism with late-onset sensorineural hearing loss; Norrie syndrome; Gernet syndrome; Jensen syndrome; Berk-Tabatznik syndrome; and Mohr-Mageroy syndrome. For each condition discussed, the author covers the ocular system involvement, the auditory system, laboratory findings, pathology, heredity, diagnosis, and prognosis. References are included in each section. 23 figures. 4 tables. 346 references.

- **Genetic Hearing Loss Associated with Integumentary Disorders**

Source: in Gorlin, R.J.; Toriello, H.V.; Cohen, M.M., Jr., eds. Hereditary Hearing Loss and Its Syndromes. New York, NY: Oxford University Press. 1995. p. 368-412.

Contact: Available from Oxford University Press. 200 Madison Avenue, New York, NY 10016. (800) 334-4249 or (212) 679-7300. Price: $195.00 plus shipping and handling. ISBN: 0195065522.

Summary: This chapter, from a text on hereditary hearing loss and its syndromes, discusses genetic hearing loss associated with integumentary disorders. The disorders discussed include Waardenburg syndrome; forelocks, backlocks, and sensorineural hearing loss; Ziprkowski-Margolis syndrome; Davenport syndrome; Woolf syndrome; Tietz-Smith syndrome; BADS and ermine phenotype; Yemenite-type hypopigmentation, blindness, and sensorineural hearing loss; universal dyschromatosis, small stature, and sensorineural hearing loss; recessive vitiligo and sensorineural hearing loss; hypopigmentation, muscle wasting, achalasia, and congenital sensorineural hearing loss; LEOPARD syndrome; multiple pigmented nevi and sensorineural hearing loss; Rapp-Hodgkin syndrome; keratitis-ichthyosis-deafness syndrome; CHIME syndrome; Desmons syndrome; Vohwinkel-Nockemann syndrome; palmoplantar hyperkeratosis and sensorineural hearing loss; Olmstead syndrome; Schwann syndrome (Bart-Pumphrey syndrome); Bjornstad syndrome; Woodhouse-Sakati syndrome; Crandall syndrome; congenital alopecia, mental retardation, and sensorineural hearing loss; DOOR syndrome; Goodman-Moghadam syndrome; Robinson syndrome; atopic dermatitis and sensorineural hearing loss; Shepard-Elliot-Mulvihill syndrome; xeroderma pigmentosum; Helweg-Larsen and Ludvigsen syndrome; cylindromatosis; Goltz-Gorlin syndrome; and Ruzicka syndrome. For each condition discussed, the author covers the clinical findings, the auditory system, craniofacial findings, the integumentary system, the vestibular system, pathology, heredity, diagnosis, and prognosis. References are included in each section. 31 figures. 1 table. 383 references.

- **Solving Skin Problems**

Source: in Touchette, N. Diabetes Problem Solver. Alexandria, VA: American Diabetes Association. 1999. p. 295-311.

Contact: Available from American Diabetes Association (ADA). Order Fulfillment Department, P.O. Box 930850, Atlanta, GA 31193-0850. (800) 232-6733. Fax (770) 442-9742. Website: www.diabetes.org. Price: $19.95 for members; plus shipping and handling. ISBN: 1570400091.

Summary: This chapter deals with solving skin problems in people who have diabetes. People who have diabetes may experience many skin problems, including digital sclerosis, Dupuytren's contracture, yellow skin, diabetic dermopathy, necrobiosis lipoidica diabeticorum, granuloma annulare, scleredema, bullosis diabeticorum, xanthomas, acanthus nigricans, vitiligo, pruritus, and necrolytic migratory erythema. Other skin problems include yeast infections; fungal infections; and bacterial infections such as impetigo, erythrasma, erysipelas, carbuncles and furuncles, cellulitis, necrotizing fascitis and cellulitis, and abscesses. In addition, skin problems may occur as a result of reactions to diabetes medications such as insulin and sulfonylureas. The chapter presents the symptoms of these skin conditions and explains what action people should take if they experience any of the symptoms of these conditions.

- **Association Between Insulin-Dependent Diabetes Mellitus and Other Autoimmune Diseases**

Source: in LeRoith, D.; Taylor, S.I.; Olefsky, J.M., eds. Diabetes Mellitus: A Fundamental and Clinical Text. Philadelphia, PA: Lippincott-Raven Publishers. 1996. p. 333-339.

Contact: Available from Lippincott-Raven Publishers. 12107 Insurance Way, Hagerstown, MD 21740-5184. (800) 777-2295. Fax (301) 824-7390. Price: $199.00. ISBN: 0397514565.

Summary: This chapter, from a medical text on diabetes mellitus, investigates the association between insulin-dependent diabetes mellitus (IDDM, or Type 1) and other autoimmune diseases. The authors first review the historical background of this autoimmune pathogenesis. Other topics include the genetics of IDDM, the genetic associations between IDDM and other autoimmune endocrinopathies, clinical relevance (notably to thyroiditis, Addison's disease, atrophic gastritis, and steroidal antibodies), and recommendations for screening. The authors conclude that IDDM often occurs in the context of other autoimmune endocrinopathies. Its most common presentation with other autoimmunity is as part of APS III, which is the constellation of IDDM and autoimmune thyroiditis, sometimes with pernicious anemia, vitiligo, and or hypogonadism. The possible genetic explanations for the association between other endocrinopathies and IDDM remain unclear. Until the issue of genetics has been resolved, the clinician must rely entirely on the recognition of subtle symptoms and a knowledge of serum autoantibody profiles to diagnose and treat polyglandular autoimmunity. 1 figure. 4 tables. 81 references.

General Home References

In addition to references for vitiligo, you may want a general home medical guide that spans all aspects of home healthcare. The following list is a recent sample of such guides (sorted alphabetically by title; hyperlinks provide rankings, information, and reviews at Amazon.com):

- **Encyclopedia of Skin and Skin Disorders (The Facts on File Library of Health and Living)** by Carol Turkington, Jeffrey S. Dover; Hardcover - 448 pages, 2nd edition (June 2002), Facts on File, Inc.; ISBN: 0816047766; http://www.amazon.com/exec/obidos/ASIN/0816047766/icongroupinterna

- **Your Skin from A to Z** by Jerome Z. Litt, M.D.; Paperback (March 2002), Barricade Books; ISBN: 1569802165; http://www.amazon.com/exec/obidos/ASIN/1569802165/icongroupinterna

- **American College of Physicians Complete Home Medical Guide (with Interactive Human Anatomy CD-ROM)** by David R. Goldmann (Editor), American College of Physicians; Hardcover - 1104 pages, Book & CD-Rom edition (1999), DK Publishing; ISBN: 0789444127; http://www.amazon.com/exec/obidos/ASIN/0789444127/icongroupinterna

- **The American Medical Association Guide to Home Caregiving** by the American Medical Association (Editor); Paperback - 256 pages 1 edition (2001), John Wiley & Sons; ISBN: 0471414093; http://www.amazon.com/exec/obidos/ASIN/0471414093/icongroupinterna

- **Anatomica : The Complete Home Medical Reference** by Peter Forrestal (Editor); Hardcover (2000), Book Sales; ISBN: 1740480309; http://www.amazon.com/exec/obidos/ASIN/1740480309/icongroupinterna

- **The HarperCollins Illustrated Medical Dictionary : The Complete Home Medical Dictionary** by Ida G. Dox, et al; Paperback - 656 pages 4th edition (2001), Harper Resource; ISBN: 0062736469; http://www.amazon.com/exec/obidos/ASIN/0062736469/icongroupinterna

- **Mayo Clinic Guide to Self-Care: Answers for Everyday Health Problems** by Philip Hagen, M.D. (Editor), et al; Paperback - 279 pages, 2nd edition (December 15, 1999), Kensington Publishing Corp.; ISBN: 0962786578; http://www.amazon.com/exec/obidos/ASIN/0962786578/icongroupinterna

- **The Merck Manual of Medical Information : Home Edition (Merck Manual of Medical Information Home Edition (Trade Paper)** by Robert

Berkow (Editor), Mark H. Beers, M.D. (Editor); Paperback - 1536 pages (2000), Pocket Books; ISBN: 0671027263;
http://www.amazon.com/exec/obidos/ASIN/0671027263/icongroupinterna

Vocabulary Builder

Anesthesia: A state characterized by loss of feeling or sensation. This depression of nerve function is usually the result of pharmacologic action and is induced to allow performance of surgery or other painful procedures. [NIH]

Aniridia: A congenital abnormality in which there is only a rudimentary iris. This is due to the failure of the optic cup to grow. Aniridia also occurs in a hereditary form, usually autosomal dominant. [NIH]

Blindness: The inability to see or the loss or absence of perception of visual stimuli. This condition may be the result of eye diseases; optic nerve diseases; optic chiasm diseases; or brain diseases affecting the visual pathways or occipital lobe. [NIH]

Carbuncle: An infection of cutaneous and subcutaneous tissue that consists of a cluster of boils. Commonly, the causative agent is staphylococcus aureus. Carbuncles produce fever, leukocytosis, extreme pain, and prostration. [NIH]

Cellulitis: An acute, diffuse, and suppurative inflammation of loose connective tissue, particularly the deep subcutaneous tissues, and sometimes muscle, which is most commonly seen as a result of infection of a wound, ulcer, or other skin lesions. [NIH]

Choroideremia: An X chromosome-linked abnormality characterized by atrophy of the choroid and degeneration of the retinal pigment epithelium causing night blindness. [NIH]

Dystrophy: Any disorder arising from defective or faulty nutrition, especially the muscular dystrophies. [EU]

Erysipelas: An acute superficial form of cellulitis involving the dermal lymphatics, usually caused by infection with group A streptococci, and chiefly characterized by a peripherally spreading hot, bright red, edematous, brawny, infiltrated, and sharply circumscribed plaque with a raised indurated border. Formerly called St. Anthony's fire. [EU]

Gastritis: Inflammation of the stomach. [EU]

Granuloma: A relatively small nodular inflammatory lesion containing grouped mononuclear phagocytes, caused by infectious and noninfectious agents. [NIH]

Heredity: 1. the genetic transmission of a particular quality or trait from parent to offspring. 2. the genetic constitution of an individual. [EU]

Hyperkeratosis: 1. hypertrophy of the corneous layer of the skin. 2a. any of various conditions marked by hyperkeratosis. 2b. a disease of cattle marked by thickening and wringling of the hide and formation of papillary outgrowths on the buccal mucous membranes, often accompanied by watery discharge from eyes and nose, diarrhoea, loss of condition, and abortion of pregnant animals, and now believed to result from ingestion of the chlorinated naphthalene of various lubricating oils. [EU]

Hypogonadism: A condition resulting from or characterized by abnormally decreased functional activity of the gonads, with retardation of growth and sexual development. [EU]

Ichthyosis: A group of cutaneous disorders characterized by increased or aberrant keratinization, resulting in noninflammatory scaling of the skin. Many different metaphors have been used to describe the appearance and texture of the skin in the various types and stages of ichthyosis, e.g. alligator, collodion, crocodile, fish, and porcupine skin. Most ichthyoses are genetically determined, while some may be acquired and develop in association with various systemic diseases or be a prominent feature in certain genetic syndromes. The term is commonly used alone to refer to i. vulgaris. [EU]

Impetigo: A common superficial bacterial infection caused by staphylococcus aureus or group A beta-hemolytic streptococci. Characteristics include pustular lesions that rupture and discharge a thin, amber-colored fluid that dries and forms a crust. This condition is commonly located on the face, especially about the mouth and nose. [NIH]

Keratitis: Inflammation of the cornea. [EU]

Myopia: That error of refraction in which rays of light entering the eye parallel to the optic axis are brought to a focus in front of the retina, as a result of the eyeball being too long from front to back (axial m.) or of an increased strength in refractive power of the media of the eye (index m.). Called also nearsightedness, because the near point is less distant than it is in emmetropia with an equal amplitude of accommodation. [EU]

Nystagmus: An involuntary, rapid, rhythmic movement of the eyeball, which may be horizontal, vertical, rotatory, or mixed, i.e., of two varieties. [EU]

Pruritus: 1. itching; an unpleasant cutaneous sensation that provokes the desire to rub or scratch the skin to obtain relief. 2. any of various conditions marked by itching, the specific site or type being indicated by a modifying term. [EU]

Retinopathy: 1. retinitis (= inflammation of the retina). 2. retinosis (=

degenerative, noninflammatory condition of the retina). [EU]

Sclerosis: A induration, or hardening; especially hardening of a part from inflammation and in diseases of the interstitial substance. The term is used chiefly for such a hardening of the nervous system due to hyperplasia of the connective tissue or to designate hardening of the blood vessels. [EU]

Transplantation: The grafting of tissues taken from the patient's own body or from another. [EU]

Vestibular: Pertaining to or toward a vestibule. In dental anatomy, used to refer to the tooth surface directed toward the vestibule of the mouth. [EU]

Xanthoma: A tumour composed of lipid-laden foam cells, which are histiocytes containing cytoplasmic lipid material. Called also xanthelasma. [EU]

CHAPTER 6. MULTIMEDIA ON VITILIGO

Overview

Information on vitiligo can come in a variety of formats. Among multimedia sources, video productions, slides, audiotapes, and computer databases are often available. In this chapter, we show you how to keep current on multimedia sources of information on vitiligo. We start with sources that have been summarized by federal agencies, and then show you how to find bibliographic information catalogued by the National Library of Medicine. If you see an interesting item, visit your local medical library to check on the availability of the title.

Bibliography: Multimedia on Vitiligo

The National Library of Medicine is a rich source of information on healthcare-related multimedia productions including slides, computer software, and databases. To access the multimedia database, go to the following Web site: **http://locatorplus.gov/**. Select "Search LOCATORplus." Once in the search area, simply type in vitiligo (or synonyms). Then, in the option box provided below the search box, select "Audiovisuals and Computer Files." From there, you can choose to sort results by publication date, author, or relevance. The following multimedia has been indexed on vitiligo. For more information, follow the hyperlink indicated:

- **Cutaneous manifestations of systemic disease.** Source: American Academy of Dermatology, and Institute for Dermatologic Communication and Education; Year: 1973; Format: Slide; [Evanston, Ill.]: The Academy, [1973]

- **Dermatoses in blacks.** Source: Georgia Regional Medical Television Network; Year: 1972; Format: Videorecording; [Atlanta: The Network; for loan or sale by Calhoun (A. W.) Medical Library, 1972]

- **Skin cancer and dermatitis factitia.** Source: Dept. of Medicine, Emory University, School of Medicine; Year: 1979; Format: Videorecording; Atlanta: Emory Medical Television Network: [for loan and sale by A. W. Calhoun Medical Library, 1979]

- **Skin diseases of the feet.** Source: Richard C. Gibbs; Year: 1973; Format: Slide; New York: Medcom, c1973

- **Vulvar disease: benign and malignant.** Source: Direction South Media; Year: 1973; Format: Filmstrip; Hunt Valley, Md.: Direction South Media, c1973

CHAPTER 7. PERIODICALS AND NEWS ON VITILIGO

Overview

Keeping up on the news relating to vitiligo can be challenging. Subscribing to targeted periodicals can be an effective way to stay abreast of recent developments on vitiligo. Periodicals include newsletters, magazines, and academic journals.

In this chapter, we suggest a number of news sources and present various periodicals that cover vitiligo beyond and including those which are published by patient associations mentioned earlier. We will first focus on news services, and then on periodicals. News services, press releases, and newsletters generally use more accessible language, so if you do chose to subscribe to one of the more technical periodicals, make sure that it uses language you can easily follow.

News Services & Press Releases

Well before articles show up in newsletters or the popular press, they may appear in the form of a press release or a public relations announcement. One of the simplest ways of tracking press releases on vitiligo is to search the news wires. News wires are used by professional journalists, and have existed since the invention of the telegraph. Today, there are several major "wires" that are used by companies, universities, and other organizations to announce new medical breakthroughs. In the following sample of sources, we will briefly describe how to access each service. These services only post recent news intended for public viewing.

PR Newswire

Perhaps the broadest of the wires is PR Newswire Association, Inc. To access this archive, simply go to **http://www.prnewswire.com**. Below the search box, select the option "The last 30 days." In the search box, type "vitiligo" or synonyms. The search results are shown by order of relevance. When reading these press releases, do not forget that the sponsor of the release may be a company or organization that is trying to sell a particular product or therapy. Their views, therefore, may be biased.

Reuters

The Reuters' Medical News database can be very useful in exploring news archives relating to vitiligo. While some of the listed articles are free to view, others can be purchased for a nominal fee. To access this archive, go to **http://www.reutershealth.com/frame2/arch.html** and search by "vitiligo" (or synonyms). The following was recently listed in this archive for vitiligo:

- **Dermal autografts for stable vitiligo may yield long-term benefits**
  Source: Reuters Medical News
  Date: September 18, 2001
  http://www.reuters.gov/archive/2001/09/18/professional/links/20010918clin008.html

- **Narrow-band UVB phototherapy effective for vitiligo**
  Source: Reuters Industry Breifing
  Date: June 28, 2001
  http://www.reuters.gov/archive/2001/06/28/business/links/20010628clin001.html

- **Adding calcipotriol to PUVA for vitiligo may hasten response**
  Source: Reuters Industry Breifing
  Date: April 10, 2001
  http://www.reuters.gov/archive/2001/04/10/business/links/20010410clin001.html

- **FDA clears PhotoMedex's excimer laser for vitiligo**
  Source: Reuters Industry Breifing
  Date: March 02, 2001
  http://www.reuters.gov/archive/2001/03/02/business/links/20010302rglt004.html

- **FDA clears PhotoMedex's excimer laser for treatment of vitiligo**
  Source: Reuters Medical News
  Date: March 02, 2001
  http://www.reuters.gov/archive/2001/03/02/professional/links/20010
  302rglt007.html

- **PhotoMedex files for expanded use of its laser system to treat vitiligo**
  Source: Reuters Industry Breifing
  Date: February 12, 2001
  http://www.reuters.gov/archive/2001/02/12/business/links/20010212
  rglt002.html

- **Long-Term Severity Of Vitiligo Can Be Predicted**
  Source: Reuters Medical News
  Date: March 05, 1998
  http://www.reuters.gov/archive/1998/03/05/professional/links/19980
  305clin009.html

The NIH

Within MEDLINEplus, the NIH has made an agreement with the New York Times Syndicate, the AP News Service, and Reuters to deliver news that can be browsed by the public. Search news releases at **http://www.nlm.nih.gov/medlineplus/alphanews_a.html.** MEDLINEplus allows you to browse across an alphabetical index. Or you can search by date at **http://www.nlm.nih.gov/medlineplus/newsbydate.html**. Often, news items are indexed by MEDLINEplus within their search engine.

Business Wire

Business Wire is similar to PR Newswire. To access this archive, simply go to **http://www.businesswire.com**. You can scan the news by industry category or company name.

Internet Wire

Internet Wire is more focused on technology than the other wires. To access this site, go to **http://www.internetwire.com** and use the "Search Archive" option. Type in "vitiligo" (or synonyms). As this service is oriented to technology, you may wish to search for press releases covering diagnostic procedures or tests that you may have read about.

Search Engines

Free-to-view news can also be found in the news section of your favorite search engines (see the health news page at Yahoo: **http://dir.yahoo.com/Health/News_and_Media/,** or use this Web site's general news search page **http://news.yahoo.com/.** Type in "vitiligo" (or synonyms). If you know the name of a company that is relevant to vitiligo, you can go to any stock trading Web site (such as **www.etrade.com**) and search for the company name there. News items across various news sources are reported on indicated hyperlinks.

BBC

Covering news from a more European perspective, the British Broadcasting Corporation (BBC) allows the public free access to their news archive located at **http://www.bbc.co.uk/.** Search by "vitiligo" (or synonyms).

Newsletter Articles

If you choose not to subscribe to a newsletter, you can nevertheless find references to newsletter articles. We recommend that you use the Combined Health Information Database, while limiting your search criteria to "newsletter articles." Again, you will need to use the "Detailed Search" option. Go directly to the following hyperlink: **http://chid.nih.gov/detail/detail.html.** Go to the bottom of the search page where "You may refine your search by." Select the dates and language that you prefer. For the format option, select "Newsletter Article."

By making these selections, and typing in "vitiligo" (or synonyms) into the "For these words:" box, you will only receive results on newsletter articles. You should check back periodically with this database as it is updated every 3 months. The following is a typical result when searching for newsletter articles on vitiligo:

- **Pseudocatalase Update**

  Source: Vitiligo Newsletter. 7(3): 8-9. August 2000.

  Contact: Available from National Vitiligo Foundation. 611 South Fleishel Avenue, Tyler, TX 75701. (903) 531-0074. Fax (903) 525-1234. E-mail: vitiligo@trimofran.org. Website: www.vitiligofoundation.org.

Summary: This newsletter article provides people who have vitiligo with information on pseudocatalase (PCAT) with calcium cream. PCAT, which is a topical prescription that inhibits the progression of pigment loss in vitiligo, works by reducing skin levels of peroxides. Increased levels of peroxides can lead to decreased activity of pigment cells. PCAT used in conjunction with a light source may result in some repigmentation. The article explains how a person who has vitiligo should use PCAT and discusses its outcomes, side effects, and stability. In addition, the article provides information on obtaining PCAT and includes a survey on PCAT use.

- **Patient Selection Is Key: Sheet Grafting Has Role in Stable Vitiligo**

Source: Skin and Allergy News. 29(2): 45. February 1998.

Summary: This newsletter article provides health professionals with information on using epidermal sheet grafting to treat vitiligo. This approach is highly effective if the disease is stable, the graft recipient area can be immobilized, and the graft itself is of appropriate and even thickness. In 20 patients treated with the procedure, 8 had 100 percent repigmentation 3 months after treatment, 2 had no response, and the remainder showed partial repigmentation, usually more than 70 percent. The poorest results occurred on the hands, eyelids, and perioral areas. The most common adverse effect was the presence of milialike cysts at the graft sites during the first 6 months after treatment.

CHAPTER 8. PHYSICIAN GUIDELINES AND DATABASES

Overview

Doctors and medical researchers rely on a number of information sources to help patients with their conditions. Many will subscribe to journals or newsletters published by their professional associations or refer to specialized textbooks or clinical guides published for the medical profession. In this chapter, we focus on databases and Internet-based guidelines created or written for this professional audience.

NIH Guidelines

For the more common diseases, The National Institutes of Health publish guidelines that are frequently consulted by physicians. Publications are typically written by one or more of the various NIH Institutes. For physician guidelines, commonly referred to as "clinical" or "professional" guidelines, you can visit the following Institutes:

- Office of the Director (OD); guidelines consolidated across agencies available at **http://www.nih.gov/health/consumer/conkey.htm**

- National Institute of General Medical Sciences (NIGMS); fact sheets available at **http://www.nigms.nih.gov/news/facts/**

- National Library of Medicine (NLM); extensive encyclopedia (A.D.A.M., Inc.) with guidelines:
  http://www.nlm.nih.gov/medlineplus/healthtopics.html

- National Institute of Arthritis and Musculoskeletal and Skin Diseases (NIAMS); fact sheets and guidelines available at
  http://www.nih.gov/niams/healthinfo/

NIH Databases

In addition to the various Institutes of Health that publish professional guidelines, the NIH has designed a number of databases for professionals.[24] Physician-oriented resources provide a wide variety of information related to the biomedical and health sciences, both past and present. The format of these resources varies. Searchable databases, bibliographic citations, full text articles (when available), archival collections, and images are all available. The following are referenced by the National Library of Medicine:[25]

- **Bioethics:** Access to published literature on the ethical, legal and public policy issues surrounding healthcare and biomedical research. This information is provided in conjunction with the Kennedy Institute of Ethics located at Georgetown University, Washington, D.C.: **http://www.nlm.nih.gov/databases/databases_bioethics.html**

- **HIV/AIDS Resources:** Describes various links and databases dedicated to HIV/AIDS research: **http://www.nlm.nih.gov/pubs/factsheets/aidsinfs.html**

- **NLM Online Exhibitions:** Describes "Exhibitions in the History of Medicine": **http://www.nlm.nih.gov/exhibition/exhibition.html**. Additional resources for historical scholarship in medicine: **http://www.nlm.nih.gov/hmd/hmd.html**

- **Biotechnology Information:** Access to public databases. The National Center for Biotechnology Information conducts research in computational biology, develops software tools for analyzing genome data, and disseminates biomedical information for the better understanding of molecular processes affecting human health and disease: **http://www.ncbi.nlm.nih.gov/**

- **Population Information:** The National Library of Medicine provides access to worldwide coverage of population, family planning, and related health issues, including family planning technology and programs, fertility, and population law and policy: **http://www.nlm.nih.gov/databases/databases_population.html**

- **Cancer Information:** Access to caner-oriented databases: **http://www.nlm.nih.gov/databases/databases_cancer.html**

---

[24] Remember, for the general public, the National Library of Medicine recommends the databases referenced in MEDLINE*plus* (**http://medlineplus.gov/** or **http://www.nlm.nih.gov/medlineplus/databases.html**).

[25] See http://www.nlm.nih.gov/databases/databases.html.

- **Profiles in Science:** Offering the archival collections of prominent twentieth-century biomedical scientists to the public through modern digital technology: **http://www.profiles.nlm.nih.gov/**

- **Chemical Information:** Provides links to various chemical databases and references: **http://sis.nlm.nih.gov/Chem/ChemMain.html**

- **Clinical Alerts:** Reports the release of findings from the NIH-funded clinical trials where such release could significantly affect morbidity and mortality: **http://www.nlm.nih.gov/databases/alerts/clinical_alerts.html**

- **Space Life Sciences:** Provides links and information to space-based research (including NASA): **http://www.nlm.nih.gov/databases/databases_space.html**

- **MEDLINE:** Bibliographic database covering the fields of medicine, nursing, dentistry, veterinary medicine, the healthcare system, and the pre-clinical sciences: **http://www.nlm.nih.gov/databases/databases_medline.html**

- **Toxicology and Environmental Health Information (TOXNET):** Databases covering toxicology and environmental health: **http://sis.nlm.nih.gov/Tox/ToxMain.html**

- **Visible Human Interface:** Anatomically detailed, three-dimensional representations of normal male and female human bodies: **http://www.nlm.nih.gov/research/visible/visible_human.html**

While all of the above references may be of interest to physicians who study and treat vitiligo, the following are particularly noteworthy.

The Combined Health Information Database

A comprehensive source of information on clinical guidelines written for professionals is the Combined Health Information Database. You will need to limit your search to "Brochure/Pamphlet," "Fact Sheet," or "Information Package" and vitiligo using the "Detailed Search" option. Go directly to the following hyperlink: **http://chid.nih.gov/detail/detail.html**. To find associations, use the drop boxes at the bottom of the search page where "You may refine your search by." For the publication date, select "All Years," select your preferred language, and the format option "Fact Sheet." By making these selections and typing "vitiligo" (or synonyms) into the "For these words:" box above, you will only receive results on fact sheets dealing with vitiligo. The following is a sample result:

- **Questions and Answers About Autoimmunity**

  Source: Bethesda, MD: National Institute of Arthritis and Musculoskeletal and Skin Diseases (NIAMS) Information Clearinghouse. 2002. 32 p.

  Contact: Available from National Institute of Arthritis and Musculoskeletal and Skin Diseases (NIAMS) Information Clearinghouse. 1 AMS Circle, Bethesda, MD 20892-3675. (877) 226-4267 toll-free or (301) 495-4484. Fax (301) 718-6366. TTY (301) 565-2966. E-mail: NIAMSInfo@mail.nih.gov. Website: www.niams.nih.gov. Price: 1 to 25 copies free. Order Number: AR-242 QA (booklet), or AR-242L QA (large print fact sheet).

  Summary: This booklet provides people who have an autoimmune disease with information on the causes, diagnosis, and treatment of such diseases. Autoimmune diseases occur when the body attacks its own cells as invaders. Although the cause of autoimmunity is unknown, most scientists believe that genetic and environmental factors are involved. Autoimmunity can affect almost any part of the body, and the problems caused by autoimmunity depend on the tissues targeted. Diagnosis is based on the medical history, a physical examination, and medical tests. Treatment depends on the type of disease and its symptoms and severity. The goals of treatment are to relieve symptoms, preserve organ function, and target disease mechanisms. The types of doctors who provide treatment for autoimmune diseases vary, and they include rheumatologists, endocrinologists, neurologists, hematologists, gastroenterologists, dermatologists, and nephrologists. Problems that people experience with an autoimmune disease also vary and may be related to self esteem, self care, family relationships, sexual relations, and pregnancy. Research is being conducted to help people with autoimmune diseases such as rheumatoid arthritis, systemic lupus erythematosus, lupus nephritis, vitiligo, type 1 diabetes, multiple sclerosis, and multiple autoimmune diseases. The booklet includes a list of government and other organizations that can provide information about autoimmunity. Appendices provide glossaries of terms and diseases.

The NLM Gateway[26]

The NLM (National Library of Medicine) Gateway is a Web-based system that lets users search simultaneously in multiple retrieval systems at the U.S. National Library of Medicine (NLM). It allows users of NLM services to initiate searches from one Web interface, providing "one-stop searching" for

---

[26] Adapted from NLM: **http://gateway.nlm.nih.gov/gw/Cmd?Overview.x**.

many of NLM's information resources or databases.[27] One target audience for the Gateway is the Internet user who is new to NLM's online resources and does not know what information is available or how best to search for it. This audience may include physicians and other healthcare providers, researchers, librarians, students, and, increasingly, patients, their families, and the public.[28] To use the NLM Gateway, simply go to the search site at **http://gateway.nlm.nih.gov/gw/Cmd**. Type "vitiligo" (or synonyms) into the search box and click "Search." The results will be presented in a tabular form, indicating the number of references in each database category.

Results Summary

Category	Items Found
Journal Articles	2329
Books / Periodicals / Audio Visual	31
Consumer Health	24
Meeting Abstracts	0
Other Collections	0
Total	2384

HSTAT[29]

HSTAT is a free, Web-based resource that provides access to full-text documents used in healthcare decision-making.[30] HSTAT's audience includes healthcare providers, health service researchers, policy makers, insurance companies, consumers, and the information professionals who serve these groups. HSTAT provides access to a wide variety of publications, including clinical practice guidelines, quick-reference guides for clinicians, consumer

---

[27] The NLM Gateway is currently being developed by the Lister Hill National Center for Biomedical Communications (LHNCBC) at the National Library of Medicine (NLM) of the National Institutes of Health (NIH).

[28] Other users may find the Gateway useful for an overall search of NLM's information resources. Some searchers may locate what they need immediately, while others will utilize the Gateway as an adjunct tool to other NLM search services such as PubMed® and MEDLINEplus®. The Gateway connects users with multiple NLM retrieval systems while also providing a search interface for its own collections. These collections include various types of information that do not logically belong in PubMed, LOCATORplus, or other established NLM retrieval systems (e.g., meeting announcements and pre-1966 journal citations). The Gateway will provide access to the information found in an increasing number of NLM retrieval systems in several phases.

[29] Adapted from HSTAT: http://www.nlm.nih.gov/pubs/factsheets/hstat.html.

[30] The HSTAT URL is **http://hstat.nlm.nih.gov/**.

health brochures, evidence reports and technology assessments from the Agency for Healthcare Research and Quality (AHRQ), as well as AHRQ's Put Prevention Into Practice.[31] Simply search by "vitiligo" (or synonyms) at the following Web site: **http://text.nlm.nih.gov**.

Coffee Break: Tutorials for Biologists[32]

Some patients may wish to have access to a general healthcare site that takes a scientific view of the news and covers recent breakthroughs in biology that may one day assist physicians in developing treatments. To this end, we recommend "Coffee Break," a collection of short reports on recent biological discoveries. Each report incorporates interactive tutorials that demonstrate how bioinformatics tools are used as a part of the research process. Currently, all Coffee Breaks are written by NCBI staff.[33] Each report is about 400 words and is usually based on a discovery reported in one or more articles from recently published, peer-reviewed literature.[34] This site has new articles every few weeks, so it can be considered an online magazine of sorts, and intended for general background information. You can access the Coffee Break Web site at **http://www.ncbi.nlm.nih.gov/Coffeebreak/**.

---

[31] Other important documents in HSTAT include: the National Institutes of Health (NIH) Consensus Conference Reports and Technology Assessment Reports; the HIV/AIDS Treatment Information Service (ATIS) resource documents; the Substance Abuse and Mental Health Services Administration's Center for Substance Abuse Treatment (SAMHSA/CSAT) Treatment Improvement Protocols (TIP) and Center for Substance Abuse Prevention (SAMHSA/CSAP) Prevention Enhancement Protocols System (PEPS); the Public Health Service (PHS) Preventive Services Task Force's *Guide to Clinical Preventive Services*; the independent, nonfederal Task Force on Community Services *Guide to Community Preventive Services*; and the Health Technology Advisory Committee (HTAC) of the Minnesota Health Care Commission (MHCC) health technology evaluations.

[32] Adapted from http://www.ncbi.nlm.nih.gov/Coffeebreak/Archive/FAQ.html.

[33] The figure that accompanies each article is frequently supplied by an expert external to NCBI, in which case the source of the figure is cited. The result is an interactive tutorial that tells a biological story.

[34] After a brief introduction that sets the work described into a broader context, the report focuses on how a molecular understanding can provide explanations of observed biology and lead to therapies for diseases. Each vignette is accompanied by a figure and hypertext links that lead to a series of pages that interactively show how NCBI tools and resources are used in the research process.

Other Commercial Databases

In addition to resources maintained by official agencies, other databases exist that are commercial ventures addressing medical professionals. Here are a few examples that may interest you:

- **CliniWeb International:** Index and table of contents to selected clinical information on the Internet; see **http://www.ohsu.edu/cliniweb/**.

- **Image Engine:** Multimedia electronic medical record system that integrates a wide range of digitized clinical images with textual data stored in the University of Pittsburgh Medical Center's MARS electronic medical record system; see the following Web site: **http://www.cml.upmc.edu/cml/imageengine/imageEngine.html**.

- **Medical World Search:** Searches full text from thousands of selected medical sites on the Internet; see **http://www.mwsearch.com/**.

- **MedWeaver:** Prototype system that allows users to search differential diagnoses for any list of signs and symptoms, to search medical literature, and to explore relevant Web sites; see **http://www.med.virginia.edu/~wmd4n/medweaver.html**.

- **Metaphrase:** Middleware component intended for use by both caregivers and medical records personnel. It converts the informal language generally used by caregivers into terms from formal, controlled vocabularies; see the following Web site: **http://www.lexical.com/Metaphrase.html**.

The Genome Project and Vitiligo

With all the discussion in the press about the Human Genome Project, it is only natural that physicians, researchers, and patients want to know about how human genes relate to vitiligo. In the following section, we will discuss databases and references used by physicians and scientists who work in this area.

Online Mendelian Inheritance in Man (OMIM)

The Online Mendelian Inheritance in Man (OMIM) database is a catalog of human genes and genetic disorders authored and edited by Dr. Victor A. McKusick and his colleagues at Johns Hopkins and elsewhere. OMIM was developed for the World Wide Web by the National Center for

Biotechnology Information (NCBI).[35] The database contains textual information, pictures, and reference information. It also contains copious links to NCBI's Entrez database of MEDLINE articles and sequence information.

Go to **http://www.ncbi.nlm.nih.gov/Omim/searchomim.html** to search the database. Type "vitiligo" (or synonyms) in the search box, and click "Submit Search." If too many results appear, you can narrow the search by adding the word "clinical." Each report will have additional links to related research and databases. By following these links, especially the link titled "Database Links," you will be exposed to numerous specialized databases that are largely used by the scientific community. These databases are overly technical and seldom used by the general public, but offer an abundance of information. The following is an example of the results you can obtain from the OMIM for vitiligo:

- **Deafness, Congenital, with Vitiligo and Achalasia**
  Web site: http://www.ncbi.nlm.nih.gov/htbin-post/Omim/dispmim?221350

- **Spastic Paraparesis, Vitiligo, Premature Graying, Characteristic Facies**
  Web site: http://www.ncbi.nlm.nih.gov/htbin-post/Omim/dispmim?270680

- **Systemic Lupus Erythematosus, Vitiligo-related**
  Web site: http://www.ncbi.nlm.nih.gov/htbin-post/Omim/dispmim?606579

- **Vitiligo**
  Web site: http://www.ncbi.nlm.nih.gov/htbin-post/Omim/dispmim?193200

- **Vitiligo, Progressive, with Mental Retardation and Urethral Duplication**
  Web site: http://www.ncbi.nlm.nih.gov/htbin-post/Omim/dispmim?277465

---

[35] Adapted from **http://www.ncbi.nlm.nih.gov/**. Established in 1988 as a national resource for molecular biology information, NCBI creates public databases, conducts research in computational biology, develops software tools for analyzing genome data, and disseminates biomedical information--all for the better understanding of molecular processes affecting human health and disease.

Genes and Disease (NCBI - Map)

The Genes and Disease database is produced by the National Center for Biotechnology Information of the National Library of Medicine at the National Institutes of Health. This Web site categorizes each disorder by the system of the body associated with it. Go to **http://www.ncbi.nlm.nih.gov/disease/**, and browse the system pages to have a full view of important conditions linked to human genes. Since this site is regularly updated, you may wish to re-visit it from time to time. The following systems and associated disorders are addressed:

- **Cancer:** Uncontrolled cell division.
  Examples: Breast And Ovarian Cancer, Burkitt lymphoma, chronic myeloid leukemia, colon cancer, lung cancer, malignant melanoma, multiple endocrine neoplasia, neurofibromatosis, p53 tumor suppressor, pancreatic cancer, prostate cancer, Ras oncogene, RB: retinoblastoma, von Hippel-Lindau syndrome.
  Web site: **http://www.ncbi.nlm.nih.gov/disease/Cancer.html**

- **Immune System:** Fights invaders.
  Examples: Asthma, autoimmune polyglandular syndrome, Crohn's disease, DiGeorge syndrome, familial Mediterranean fever, immunodeficiency with Hyper-IgM, severe combined immunodeficiency.
  Web site: **http://www.ncbi.nlm.nih.gov/disease/Immune.html**

- **Metabolism:** Food and energy.
  Examples: Adreno-leukodystrophy, Atherosclerosis, Best disease, Gaucher disease, Glucose galactose malabsorption, Gyrate atrophy, Juvenile onset diabetes, Obesity, Paroxysmal nocturnal hemoglobinuria, Phenylketonuria, Refsum disease, Tangier disease, Tay-Sachs disease.
  Web site: **http://www.ncbi.nlm.nih.gov/disease/Metabolism.html**

- **Muscle and Bone:** Movement and growth.
  Examples: Duchenne muscular dystrophy, Ellis-van Creveld syndrome, Marfan syndrome, myotonic dystrophy, spinal muscular atrophy.
  Web site: **http://www.ncbi.nlm.nih.gov/disease/Muscle.html**

- **Nervous System:** Mind and body.
  Examples: Alzheimer disease, Amyotrophic lateral sclerosis, Angelman syndrome, Charcot-Marie-Tooth disease, epilepsy, essential tremor, Fragile X syndrome, Friedreich's ataxia, Huntington disease, Niemann-Pick disease, Parkinson disease, Prader-Willi syndrome, Rett syndrome, Spinocerebellar atrophy, Williams syndrome.
  Web site: **http://www.ncbi.nlm.nih.gov/disease/Brain.html**

- **Signals:** Cellular messages.
  Examples: Ataxia telangiectasia, Baldness, Cockayne syndrome, Glaucoma, SRY: sex determination, Tuberous sclerosis, Waardenburg syndrome, Werner syndrome.
  Web site: **http://www.ncbi.nlm.nih.gov/disease/Signals.html**

- **Transporters:** Pumps and channels.
  Examples: Cystic Fibrosis, deafness, diastrophic dysplasia, Hemophilia A, long-QT syndrome, Menkes syndrome, Pendred syndrome, polycystic kidney disease, sickle cell anemia, Wilson's disease, Zellweger syndrome.
  Web site: **http://www.ncbi.nlm.nih.gov/disease/Transporters.html**

Entrez

Entrez is a search and retrieval system that integrates several linked databases at the National Center for Biotechnology Information (NCBI). These databases include nucleotide sequences, protein sequences, macromolecular structures, whole genomes, and MEDLINE through PubMed. Entrez provides access to the following databases:

- **PubMed:** Biomedical literature (PubMed),
  Web site: **http://www.ncbi.nlm.nih.gov/entrez/query.fcgi?db=PubMed**

- **Nucleotide Sequence Database (Genbank):**
  Web site:
  http://www.ncbi.nlm.nih.gov/entrez/query.fcgi?db=Nucleotide

- **Protein Sequence Database:**
  Web site: **http://www.ncbi.nlm.nih.gov/entrez/query.fcgi?db=Protein**

- **Structure:** Three-dimensional macromolecular structures,
  Web site: **http://www.ncbi.nlm.nih.gov/entrez/query.fcgi?db=Structure**

- **Genome:** Complete genome assemblies,
  Web site: **http://www.ncbi.nlm.nih.gov/entrez/query.fcgi?db=Genome**

- **PopSet:** Population study data sets,
  Web site: **http://www.ncbi.nlm.nih.gov/entrez/query.fcgi?db=Popset**

- **OMIM:** Online Mendelian Inheritance in Man,
  Web site: **http://www.ncbi.nlm.nih.gov/entrez/query.fcgi?db=OMIM**

- **Taxonomy:** Organisms in GenBank,
  Web site:
  http://www.ncbi.nlm.nih.gov/entrez/query.fcgi?db=Taxonomy

- **Books:** Online books,
  Web site: **http://www.ncbi.nlm.nih.gov/entrez/query.fcgi?db=books**

- **ProbeSet:** Gene Expression Omnibus (GEO),
  Web site: **http://www.ncbi.nlm.nih.gov/entrez/query.fcgi?db=geo**

- **3D Domains:** Domains from Entrez Structure,
  Web site: **http://www.ncbi.nlm.nih.gov/entrez/query.fcgi?db=geo**

- **NCBI's Protein Sequence Information Survey Results:**
  Web site: **http://www.ncbi.nlm.nih.gov/About/proteinsurvey/**

To access the Entrez system at the National Center for Biotechnology Information, go to **http://www.ncbi.nlm.nih.gov/entrez**, and then select the database that you would like to search. The databases available are listed in the drop box next to "Search." In the box next to "for," enter "vitiligo" (or synonyms) and click "Go."

Jablonski's Multiple Congenital Anomaly/Mental Retardation (MCA/MR) Syndromes Database[36]

This online resource can be quite useful. It has been developed to facilitate the identification and differentiation of syndromic entities. Special attention is given to the type of information that is usually limited or completely omitted in existing reference sources due to space limitations of the printed form.

At **http://www.nlm.nih.gov/mesh/jablonski/syndrome_toc/toc_a.html** you can also search across syndromes using an alphabetical index. You can also search at **http://www.nlm.nih.gov/mesh/jablonski/syndrome_db.html**.

The Genome Database[37]

Established at Johns Hopkins University in Baltimore, Maryland in 1990, the Genome Database (GDB) is the official central repository for genomic mapping data resulting from the Human Genome Initiative. In the spring of 1999, the Bioinformatics Supercomputing Centre (BiSC) at the Hospital for Sick Children in Toronto, Ontario assumed the management of GDB. The Human Genome Initiative is a worldwide research effort focusing on structural analysis of human DNA to determine the location and sequence of the estimated 100,000 human genes. In support of this project, GDB stores

---

[36] Adapted from the National Library of Medicine:
http://www.nlm.nih.gov/mesh/jablonski/about_syndrome.html.
[37] Adapted from the Genome Database:
http://gdbwww.gdb.org/gdb/aboutGDB.html#mission.

and curates data generated by researchers worldwide who are engaged in the mapping effort of the Human Genome Project (HGP). GDB's mission is to provide scientists with an encyclopedia of the human genome which is continually revised and updated to reflect the current state of scientific knowledge. Although GDB has historically focused on gene mapping, its focus will broaden as the Genome Project moves from mapping to sequence, and finally, to functional analysis.

To access the GDB, simply go to the following hyperlink: **http://www.gdb.org/**. Search "All Biological Data" by "Keyword." Type "vitiligo" (or synonyms) into the search box, and review the results. If more than one word is used in the search box, then separate each one with the word "and" or "or" (using "or" might be useful when using synonyms). This database is extremely technical as it was created for specialists. The articles are the results which are the most accessible to non-professionals and often listed under the heading "Citations." The contact names are also accessible to non-professionals.

Specialized References

The following books are specialized references written for professionals interested in vitiligo (sorted alphabetically by title, hyperlinks provide rankings, information, and reviews at Amazon.com):

- **Atlas of Clinical Dermatology** by Du Vivier; Hardcover, 3rd edition (June 3, 2002), Churchill Livingstone; ISBN: 0443072205; **http://www.amazon.com/exec/obidos/ASIN/0443072205/icongroupinterna**

- **Clinical Dermatology** by John A. Hunter, et al; Paperback, 3rd edition (June 2002), Blackwell Science Inc; ISBN: 0632059168; **http://www.amazon.com/exec/obidos/ASIN/0632059168/icongroupinterna**

- **Clinical Dermatology: A Color Guide to Diagnosis and Therapy** by Thomas P. Habif; Hardcover, 4th edition (July 15, 2002), Mosby-Year Book; ISBN: 0323013198; **http://www.amazon.com/exec/obidos/ASIN/0323013198/icongroupinterna**

- **Common Skin Diseases** by Thomas F. Poyner; Paperback - 176 pages, 1st edition (March 15, 2000), Blackwell Science Inc.; ISBN: 0632051345; **http://www.amazon.com/exec/obidos/ASIN/0071054480/icongroupinterna**

- **Dermatology (Pocket Brain)** by Kimberly N. Jones; Hardcover (March 2002); ISBN: 0967783925; **http://www.amazon.com/exec/obidos/ASIN/0967783925/icongroupinterna**

- **Dermatology for Clinicians** by Massad G. Joseph; Hardcover - 320 pages (June 5, 2002), CRC Press-Parthenon Publishers; ISBN: 1842141260; http://www.amazon.com/exec/obidos/ASIN/1842141260/icongroupinterna

- **Essential Dermatopathology** by Ronald P. Rapini; Hardcover (August 2002), Mosby-Year Book; ISBN: 0323011985; http://www.amazon.com/exec/obidos/ASIN/0323011985/icongroupinterna

- **Evidence-Based Dermatology** by Maibach; Hardcover (March 2002), B C Decker; ISBN: 1550091727; http://www.amazon.com/exec/obidos/ASIN/1550091727/icongroupinterna

- **A Multi-Cultural Atlas of Skin Conditions** by Darya Samolis, Yuri N. Perjamutrov; Paperback - 120 pages (March 19, 2002); ISBN: 1873413424; http://www.amazon.com/exec/obidos/ASIN/1873413424/icongroupinterna

- **Treatment of Skin Disease** by Mark Lebwohl, et al; Hardcover - 600 pages, 1st edition (March 27, 2002), Mosby, Inc.; ISBN: 0723431981; http://www.amazon.com/exec/obidos/ASIN/0723431981/icongroupinterna

Vocabulary Builder

Nephritis: Inflammation of the kidney; a focal or diffuse proliferative or destructive process which may involve the glomerulus, tubule, or interstitial renal tissue. [EU]

Paraparesis: Mild to moderate loss of bilateral lower extremity motor function, which may be a manifestation of spinal cord diseases; peripheral nervous system diseases; muscular diseases; intracranial hypertension; parasagittal brain lesions; and other conditions. [NIH]

Spastic: 1. of the nature of or characterized by spasms. 2. hypertonic, so that the muscles are stiff and the movements awkward. 3. a person exhibiting spasticity, such as occurs in spastic paralysis or in cerebral palsy. [EU]

CHAPTER 9. DISSERTATIONS ON VITILIGO

Overview

University researchers are active in studying almost all known diseases. The result of research is often published in the form of Doctoral or Master's dissertations. You should understand, therefore, that applied diagnostic procedures and/or therapies can take many years to develop after the thesis that proposed the new technique or approach was written.

In this chapter, we will give you a bibliography on recent dissertations relating to vitiligo. You can read about these in more detail using the Internet or your local medical library. We will also provide you with information on how to use the Internet to stay current on dissertations.

Dissertations on Vitiligo

ProQuest Digital Dissertations is the largest archive of academic dissertations available. From this archive, we have compiled the following list covering dissertations devoted to vitiligo. You will see that the information provided includes the dissertation's title, its author, and the author's institution. To read more about the following, simply use the Internet address indicated. The following covers recent dissertations dealing with vitiligo:

- **Alopecia and Vitiligo in Autoimmune Polyendocrine Syndrome Type I** by Hedstrand, Hakan Olov; Phd from Uppsala Universitet (sweden), 2000, 44 pages
  http://wwwlib.umi.com/dissertations/fullcit/f1169505

Keeping Current

As previously mentioned, an effective way to stay current on dissertations dedicated to vitiligo is to use the database called *ProQuest Digital Dissertations* via the Internet, located at the following Web address: **http://wwwlib.umi.com/dissertations.** The site allows you to freely access the last two years of citations and abstracts. Ask your medical librarian if the library has full and unlimited access to this database. From the library, you should be able to do more complete searches than with the limited 2-year access available to the general public.

PART III. APPENDICES

ABOUT PART III

Part III is a collection of appendices on general medical topics which may be of interest to patients with vitiligo and related conditions.

APPENDIX A. RESEARCHING YOUR MEDICATIONS

Overview

There are a number of sources available on new or existing medications which could be prescribed to patients with vitiligo. While a number of hard copy or CD-Rom resources are available to patients and physicians for research purposes, a more flexible method is to use Internet-based databases. In this chapter, we will begin with a general overview of medications. We will then proceed to outline official recommendations on how you should view your medications. You may also want to research medications that you are currently taking for other conditions as they may interact with medications for vitiligo. Research can give you information on the side effects, interactions, and limitations of prescription drugs used in the treatment of vitiligo. Broadly speaking, there are two sources of information on approved medications: public sources and private sources. We will emphasize free-to-use public sources.

Your Medications: The Basics[38]

The Agency for Health Care Research and Quality has published extremely useful guidelines on how you can best participate in the medication aspects of vitiligo. Taking medicines is not always as simple as swallowing a pill. It can involve many steps and decisions each day. The AHCRQ recommends that patients with vitiligo take part in treatment decisions. Do not be afraid to ask questions and talk about your concerns. By taking a moment to ask questions early, you may avoid problems later. Here are some points to cover each time a new medicine is prescribed:

- Ask about all parts of your treatment, including diet changes, exercise, and medicines.

- Ask about the risks and benefits of each medicine or other treatment you might receive.

- Ask how often you or your doctor will check for side effects from a given medication.

Do not hesitate to ask what is important to you about your medicines. You may want a medicine with the fewest side effects, or the fewest doses to take each day. You may care most about cost, or how the medicine might affect how you live or work. Or, you may want the medicine your doctor believes will work the best. Telling your doctor will help him or her select the best treatment for you.

Do not be afraid to "bother" your doctor with your concerns and questions about medications for vitiligo. You can also talk to a nurse or a pharmacist. They can help you better understand your treatment plan. Feel free to bring a friend or family member with you when you visit your doctor. Talking over your options with someone you trust can help you make better choices, especially if you are not feeling well. Specifically, ask your doctor the following:

- The name of the medicine and what it is supposed to do.

- How and when to take the medicine, how much to take, and for how long.

- What food, drinks, other medicines, or activities you should avoid while taking the medicine.

- What side effects the medicine may have, and what to do if they occur.

- If you can get a refill, and how often.

---

[38] This section is adapted from AHCRQ: **http://www.ahcpr.gov/consumer/ncpiebro.htm**.

- About any terms or directions you do not understand.

- What to do if you miss a dose.

- If there is written information you can take home (most pharmacies have information sheets on your prescription medicines; some even offer large-print or Spanish versions).

Do not forget to tell your doctor about all the medicines you are currently taking (not just those for vitiligo). This includes prescription medicines and the medicines that you buy over the counter. Then your doctor can avoid giving you a new medicine that may not work well with the medications you take now. When talking to your doctor, you may wish to prepare a list of medicines you currently take, the reason you take them, and how you take them. Be sure to include the following information for each:

- Name of medicine

- Reason taken

- Dosage

- Time(s) of day

Also include any over-the-counter medicines, such as:

- Laxatives

- Diet pills

- Vitamins

- Cold medicine

- Aspirin or other pain, headache, or fever medicine

- Cough medicine

- Allergy relief medicine

- Antacids

- Sleeping pills

- Others (include names)

Learning More about Your Medications

Because of historical investments by various organizations and the emergence of the Internet, it has become rather simple to learn about the medications your doctor has recommended for vitiligo. One such source is the United States Pharmacopeia. In 1820, eleven physicians met in Washington, D.C. to establish the first compendium of standard drugs for the United States. They called this compendium the "U.S. Pharmacopeia (USP)." Today, the USP is a non-profit organization consisting of 800 volunteer scientists, eleven elected officials, and 400 representatives of state associations and colleges of medicine and pharmacy. The USP is located in Rockville, Maryland, and its home page is located at **www.usp.org**. The USP currently provides standards for over 3,700 médications. The resulting USP DI® Advice for the Patient® can be accessed through the National Library of Medicine of the National Institutes of Health. The database is partially derived from lists of federally approved medications in the Food and Drug Administration's (FDA) Drug Approvals database.[39]

While the FDA database is rather large and difficult to navigate, the Phamacopeia is both user-friendly and free to use. It covers more than 9,000 prescription and over-the-counter medications. To access this database, simply type the following hyperlink into your Web browser: **http://www.nlm.nih.gov/medlineplus/druginformation.html**. To view examples of a given medication (brand names, category, description, preparation, proper use, precautions, side effects, etc.), simply follow the hyperlinks indicated within the United States Pharmacopoeia. It is important to read the disclaimer by the United States Pharmacopoeia (**http://www.nlm.nih.gov/medlineplus/drugdisclaimer.html**) before using the information provided.

Of course, we as editors cannot be certain as to what medications you are taking. Therefore, we have compiled a list of medications associated with the treatment of vitiligo. Once again, due to space limitations, we only list a sample of medications and provide hyperlinks to ample documentation (e.g. typical dosage, side effects, drug-interaction risks, etc.). The following drugs have been mentioned in the Pharmacopeia and other sources as being potentially applicable to vitiligo:

Chloroquine

- **Systemic - U.S. Brands:** Aralen
  http://www.nlm.nih.gov/medlineplus/druginfo/chloroquinesyst emic202133.html

---

Methoxsalen

- **Systemic - U.S. Brands:** 8-MOP; Oxsoralen-Ultra
  http://www.nlm.nih.gov/medlineplus/druginfo/methoxsalensys
  temic202357.html

Nadroparin

- **Systemic - U.S. Brands:**
  http://www.nlm.nih.gov/medlineplus/druginfo/chloroquinesyst
  emic202133.html

Nafarelin

- **Systemic - U.S. Brands:** Synarel
  http://www.nlm.nih.gov/medlineplus/druginfo/nafarelinsystem
  ic202646.html

Naltrexone

- **Systemic - U.S. Brands:** ReVia
  http://www.nlm.nih.gov/medlineplus/druginfo/naltrexonesyste
  mic202388.html

Naphazoline

- **Ophthalmic - U.S. Brands:** Ak-Con; Albalon; Allerest; I-Naphline;
  Nafazair; Naphcon; VasoClear
  http://www.nlm.nih.gov/medlineplus/druginfo/naphazolineoph
  thalmic202389.html

Naratriptan

- **Systemic - U.S. Brands:** Amerge
  http://www.nlm.nih.gov/medlineplus/druginfo/naratriptansyste
  mic203513.html

Narcotic Analgesics and Acetaminophen

- **Systemic - U.S. Brands:** Allay; Anexsia 5/500; Anexsia 7.5/650;
  Anolor DH 5; Bancap-HC; Capital with Codeine; Co-Gesic;
  Darvocet-N 100; Darvocet-N 50; DHCplus; Dolacet; Dolagesic;
  Duocet; E-Lor; Endocet; EZ III; Hycomed; Hyco-Pap; Hydrocet;
  Hydrogesic; HY-PHEN; Lorcet 10/650; L
  http://www.nlm.nih.gov/medlineplus/druginfo/narcoticanalgesi
  csandacetamino202392.html

Narcotic Analgesics and Aspirin

- **Systemic - U.S. Brands:** Damason-P; Darvon Compound-65; Empirin with Codeine No.3; Empirin with Codeine No.4; Endodan; Lortab ASA; Panasal 5/500; PC-Cap; Percodan; Percodan-Demi; Propoxyphene Compound-65; Roxiprin; Synalgos-DC; Talwin Compound
  http://www.nlm.nih.gov/medlineplus/druginfo/narcoticanalgesi
  csandaspirinsy202393.html

Narcotic Analgesics for Pain Relief

- **Systemic - U.S. Brands:** Astramorph PF; Buprenex; Cotanal-65; Darvon; Darvon-N; Demerol; Dilaudid; Dilaudid-5; Dilaudid-HP; Dolophine; Duramorph; Hydrostat IR; Kadian; Levo-Dromoran; M S Contin; Methadose; MS/L; MS/L Concentrate; MS/S; MSIR; Nubain; Numorphan; OMS Concentrate;
  http://www.nlm.nih.gov/medlineplus/druginfo/narcoticanalgesi
  csforpainrelie202390.html

Narcotic Analgesics for Surgery and Obstetrics

- **Systemic - U.S. Brands:** Alfenta; Astramorph; Astramorph PF; Buprenex; Demerol; Duramorph; Nubain; Stadol; Sublimaze; Sufenta; Ultiva
  http://www.nlm.nih.gov/medlineplus/druginfo/narcoticanalgesi
  csforsurgeryan202391.html

Natamycin

- **Ophthalmic - U.S. Brands:** Natacyn
  http://www.nlm.nih.gov/medlineplus/druginfo/natamycinophth
  almic202394.html

Nateglinide

- **Systemic - U.S. Brands:** Starlix
  http://www.nlm.nih.gov/medlineplus/druginfo/nateglinidesyste
  mic500277.html

Commercial Databases

In addition to the medications listed in the USP above, a number of commercial sites are available by subscription to physicians and their institutions. You may be able to access these sources from your local medical library or your doctor's office.

Reuters Health Drug Database

The Reuters Health Drug Database can be searched by keyword at the hyperlink: **http://www.reutershealth.com/frame2/drug.html**. The following medications are listed in the Reuters' database as associated with vitiligo (including those with contraindications):[40]

- **Capsaicin**
  http://www.reutershealth.com/atoz/html/Capsaicin.htm

- **Didanosine**
  http://www.reutershealth.com/atoz/html/Didanosine.htm

- **Didanosine (ddl; dideoxyinosine)**
  http://www.reutershealth.com/atoz/html/Didanosine_(ddl;_dideoxyinosine).htm

Mosby's GenRx

Mosby's GenRx database (also available on CD-Rom and book format) covers 45,000 drug products including generics and international brands. It provides prescribing information, drug interactions, and patient information. Information in Mosby's GenRx database can be obtained at the following hyperlink: **http://www.genrx.com/Mosby/PhyGenRx/group.html**.

Physicians Desk Reference

The Physicians Desk Reference database (also available in CD-Rom and book format) is a full-text drug database. The database is searchable by brand name, generic name or by indication. It features multiple drug interactions reports. Information can be obtained at the following hyperlink: **http://physician.pdr.net/physician/templates/en/acl/psuser_t.htm**.

---

[40] Adapted from *A to Z Drug Facts* by Facts and Comparisons.

Other Web Sites

A number of additional Web sites discuss drug information. As an example, you may like to look at **www.drugs.com** which reproduces the information in the Pharmacopeia as well as commercial information. You may also want to consider the Web site of the Medical Letter, Inc. which allows users to download articles on various drugs and therapeutics for a nominal fee: http://www.medletter.com/.

Contraindications and Interactions (Hidden Dangers)

Some of the medications mentioned in the previous discussions can be problematic for patients with vitiligo--not because they are used in the treatment process, but because of contraindications, or side effects. Medications with contraindications are those that could react with drugs used to treat vitiligo or potentially create deleterious side effects in patients with vitiligo. You should ask your physician about any contraindications, especially as these might apply to other medications that you may be taking for common ailments.

Drug-drug interactions occur when two or more drugs react with each other. This drug-drug interaction may cause you to experience an unexpected side effect. Drug interactions may make your medications less effective, cause unexpected side effects, or increase the action of a particular drug. Some drug interactions can even be harmful to you.

Be sure to read the label every time you use a nonprescription or prescription drug, and take the time to learn about drug interactions. These precautions may be critical to your health. You can reduce the risk of potentially harmful drug interactions and side effects with a little bit of knowledge and common sense.

Drug labels contain important information about ingredients, uses, warnings, and directions which you should take the time to read and understand. Labels also include warnings about possible drug interactions. Further, drug labels may change as new information becomes available. This is why it's especially important to read the label every time you use a medication. When your doctor prescribes a new drug, discuss all over-the-counter and prescription medications, dietary supplements, vitamins, botanicals, minerals and herbals you take as well as the foods you eat. Ask your pharmacist for the package insert for each prescription drug you take.

The package insert provides more information about potential drug interactions.

A Final Warning

At some point, you may hear of alternative medications from friends, relatives, or in the news media. Advertisements may suggest that certain alternative drugs can produce positive results for patients with vitiligo. Exercise caution--some of these drugs may have fraudulent claims, and others may actually hurt you. The Food and Drug Administration (FDA) is the official U.S. agency charged with discovering which medications are likely to improve the health of patients with vitiligo. The FDA warns patients to watch out for[41]:

- Secret formulas (real scientists share what they know)

- Amazing breakthroughs or miracle cures (real breakthroughs don't happen very often; when they do, real scientists do not call them amazing or miracles)

- Quick, painless, or guaranteed cures

- If it sounds too good to be true, it probably isn't true.

If you have any questions about any kind of medical treatment, the FDA may have an office near you. Look for their number in the blue pages of the phone book. You can also contact the FDA through its toll-free number, 1-888-INFO-FDA (1-888-463-6332), or on the World Wide Web at **www.fda.gov**.

General References

In addition to the resources provided earlier in this chapter, the following general references describe medications (sorted alphabetically by title; hyperlinks provide rankings, information and reviews at Amazon.com):

- **Comprehensive Dermatologic Drug Therapy** by Stephen E. Wolverton (Editor); Paperback - 656 pages (March 15, 2001), W B Saunders Co; ISBN: 0721677282;
  http://www.amazon.com/exec/obidos/ASIN/0721677282/icongroupinterna

---

[41] This section has been adapted from http://www.fda.gov/opacom/lowlit/medfraud.html.

- **Drug Eruption Reference Manual 2000, Millennium Edition** by Jerome Z. Litt, M.D. (Editor); Paperback - 662 pages (April 15, 2000), Parthenon Pub Group; ISBN: 185070788X;
http://www.amazon.com/exec/obidos/ASIN/185070788X/icongroupinterna

- **Pocket Guide to Medications Used in Dermatology** by Andrew J. Scheman, David L. Severson; Paperback - 230 pages, 6th edition (June 15, 1999), Lippincott Williams & Wilkins Publishers; ISBN: 0781721008;
http://www.amazon.com/exec/obidos/ASIN/0781721008/icongroupinterna

- **Complete Guide to Prescription and Nonprescription Drugs 2001 (Complete Guide to Prescription and Nonprescription Drugs, 2001)** by H. Winter Griffith, Paperback 16th edition (2001), Medical Surveillance; ISBN: 0942447417;
http://www.amazon.com/exec/obidos/ASIN/039952634X/icongroupinterna

- **The Essential Guide to Prescription Drugs, 2001** by James J. Rybacki, James W. Long; Paperback - 1274 pages (2001), Harper Resource; ISBN: 0060958162;
http://www.amazon.com/exec/obidos/ASIN/0060958162/icongroupinterna

- **Handbook of Commonly Prescribed Drugs** by G. John Digregorio, Edward J. Barbieri; Paperback 16th edition (2001), Medical Surveillance; ISBN: 0942447417;
http://www.amazon.com/exec/obidos/ASIN/0942447417/icongroupinterna

- **Johns Hopkins Complete Home Encyclopedia of Drugs 2nd ed.** by Simeon Margolis (Ed.), Johns Hopkins; Hardcover - 835 pages (2000), Rebus; ISBN: 0929661583;
http://www.amazon.com/exec/obidos/ASIN/0929661583/icongroupinterna

- **Medical Pocket Reference: Drugs 2002** by Springhouse Paperback 1st edition (2001), Lippincott Williams & Wilkins Publishers; ISBN: 1582550964;
http://www.amazon.com/exec/obidos/ASIN/1582550964/icongroupinterna

- **PDR** by Medical Economics Staff, Medical Economics Staff Hardcover - 3506 pages 55th edition (2000), Medical Economics Company; ISBN: 1563633752;
http://www.amazon.com/exec/obidos/ASIN/1563633752/icongroupinterna

- **Pharmacy Simplified: A Glossary of Terms** by James Grogan; Paperback - 432 pages, 1st edition (2001), Delmar Publishers; ISBN: 0766828581;
http://www.amazon.com/exec/obidos/ASIN/0766828581/icongroupinterna

- **Physician Federal Desk Reference** by Christine B. Fraizer; Paperback 2nd edition (2001), Medicode Inc; ISBN: 1563373971;
http://www.amazon.com/exec/obidos/ASIN/1563373971/icongroupinterna

- **Physician's Desk Reference Supplements** Paperback - 300 pages, 53 edition (1999), ISBN: 1563632950;
http://www.amazon.com/exec/obidos/ASIN/1563632950/icongroupinterna

Vocabulary Builder

The following vocabulary builder gives definitions of words used in this chapter that have not been defined in previous chapters:

Analgesic: An agent that alleviates pain without causing loss of consciousness. [EU]

Chloroquine: The prototypical antimalarial agent with a mechanism that is not well understood. It has also been used to treat rheumatoid arthritis, systemic lupus erythematosus, and in the systemic therapy of amebic liver abscesses. [NIH]

Codeine: An opioid analgesic related to morphine but with less potent analgesic properties and mild sedative effects. It also acts centrally to suppress cough. [NIH]

Didanosine: A dideoxynucleoside compound in which the 3'-hydroxy group on the sugar moiety has been replaced by a hydrogen. This modification prevents the formation of phosphodiester linkages which are needed for the completion of nucleic acid chains. Didanosine is a potent inhibitor of HIV replication, acting as a chain-terminator of viral DNA by binding to reverse transcriptase; ddI is then metabolized to dideoxyadenosine triphosphate, its putative active metabolite. [NIH]

Methoxsalen: A naturally occurring furocoumarin compound found in several species of plants, including Psoralea corylifolia. It is a photoactive substance that forms DNA adducts in the presence of ultraviolet A irradiation. [NIH]

Naltrexone: Derivative of noroxymorphone that is the N-cyclopropylmethyl congener of naloxone. It is a narcotic antagonist that is effective orally, longer lasting and more potent than naloxone, and has been proposed for the treatment of heroin addiction. The FDA has approved naltrexone for the treatment of alcohol dependence. [NIH]

Naphazoline: An adrenergic vasoconstrictor agent used as a decongestant. [NIH]

Natamycin: Amphoteric macrolide antifungal antibiotic from Streptomyces natalensis or S. chattanoogensis. It is used for a variety of fungal infections, mainly topically. [NIH]

Propoxyphene: A narcotic analgesic structurally related to methadone. Only the dextro-isomer has an analgesic effect; the levo-isomer appears to exert an antitussive effect. [NIH]

APPENDIX B. RESEARCHING ALTERNATIVE MEDICINE

Overview

Complementary and alternative medicine (CAM) is one of the most contentious aspects of modern medical practice. You may have heard of these treatments on the radio or on television. Maybe you have seen articles written about these treatments in magazines, newspapers, or books. Perhaps your friends or doctor have mentioned alternatives.

In this chapter, we will begin by giving you a broad perspective on complementary and alternative therapies. Next, we will introduce you to official information sources on CAM relating to vitiligo. Finally, at the conclusion of this chapter, we will provide a list of readings on vitiligo from various authors. We will begin, however, with the National Center for Complementary and Alternative Medicine's (NCCAM) overview of complementary and alternative medicine.

What Is CAM?[42]

Complementary and alternative medicine (CAM) covers a broad range of healing philosophies, approaches, and therapies. Generally, it is defined as those treatments and healthcare practices which are not taught in medical schools, used in hospitals, or reimbursed by medical insurance companies. Many CAM therapies are termed "holistic," which generally means that the healthcare practitioner considers the whole person, including physical, mental, emotional, and spiritual health. Some of these therapies are also known as "preventive," which means that the practitioner educates and

---

[42] Adapted from the NCCAM: **http://nccam.nih.gov/nccam/fcp/faq/index.html#what-is**.

treats the person to prevent health problems from arising, rather than treating symptoms after problems have occurred.

People use CAM treatments and therapies in a variety of ways. Therapies are used alone (often referred to as alternative), in combination with other alternative therapies, or in addition to conventional treatment (sometimes referred to as complementary). Complementary and alternative medicine, or "integrative medicine," includes a broad range of healing philosophies, approaches, and therapies. Some approaches are consistent with physiological principles of Western medicine, while others constitute healing systems with non-Western origins. While some therapies are far outside the realm of accepted Western medical theory and practice, others are becoming established in mainstream medicine.

Complementary and alternative therapies are used in an effort to prevent illness, reduce stress, prevent or reduce side effects and symptoms, or control or cure disease. Some commonly used methods of complementary or alternative therapy include mind/body control interventions such as visualization and relaxation, manual healing including acupressure and massage, homeopathy, vitamins or herbal products, and acupuncture.

What Are the Domains of Alternative Medicine?[43]

The list of CAM practices changes continually. The reason being is that these new practices and therapies are often proved to be safe and effective, and therefore become generally accepted as "mainstream" healthcare practices. Today, CAM practices may be grouped within five major domains: (1) alternative medical systems, (2) mind-body interventions, (3) biologically-based treatments, (4) manipulative and body-based methods, and (5) energy therapies. The individual systems and treatments comprising these categories are too numerous to list in this sourcebook. Thus, only limited examples are provided within each.

Alternative Medical Systems

Alternative medical systems involve complete systems of theory and practice that have evolved independent of, and often prior to, conventional biomedical approaches. Many are traditional systems of medicine that are

---

[43] Adapted from the NCCAM: http://nccam.nih.gov/nccam/fcp/classify/index.html.

practiced by individual cultures throughout the world, including a number of venerable Asian approaches.

Traditional oriental medicine emphasizes the balance or disturbances of qi (pronounced chi) or vital energy in health and disease, respectively. Traditional oriental medicine consists of a group of techniques and methods including acupuncture, herbal medicine, oriental massage, and qi gong (a form of energy therapy). Acupuncture involves stimulating specific anatomic points in the body for therapeutic purposes, usually by puncturing the skin with a thin needle.

Ayurveda is India's traditional system of medicine. Ayurvedic medicine (meaning "science of life") is a comprehensive system of medicine that places equal emphasis on body, mind, and spirit. Ayurveda strives to restore the innate harmony of the individual. Some of the primary Ayurvedic treatments include diet, exercise, meditation, herbs, massage, exposure to sunlight, and controlled breathing.

Other traditional healing systems have been developed by the world's indigenous populations. These populations include Native American, Aboriginal, African, Middle Eastern, Tibetan, and Central and South American cultures. Homeopathy and naturopathy are also examples of complete alternative medicine systems.

Homeopathic medicine is an unconventional Western system that is based on the principle that "like cures like," i.e., that the same substance that in large doses produces the symptoms of an illness, in very minute doses cures it. Homeopathic health practitioners believe that the more dilute the remedy, the greater its potency. Therefore, they use small doses of specially prepared plant extracts and minerals to stimulate the body's defense mechanisms and healing processes in order to treat illness.

Naturopathic medicine is based on the theory that disease is a manifestation of alterations in the processes by which the body naturally heals itself and emphasizes health restoration rather than disease treatment. Naturopathic physicians employ an array of healing practices, including the following: diet and clinical nutrition, homeopathy, acupuncture, herbal medicine, hydrotherapy (the use of water in a range of temperatures and methods of applications), spinal and soft-tissue manipulation, physical therapies (such as those involving electrical currents, ultrasound, and light), therapeutic counseling, and pharmacology.

Mind-Body Interventions

Mind-body interventions employ a variety of techniques designed to facilitate the mind's capacity to affect bodily function and symptoms. Only a select group of mind-body interventions having well-documented theoretical foundations are considered CAM. For example, patient education and cognitive-behavioral approaches are now considered "mainstream." On the other hand, complementary and alternative medicine includes meditation, certain uses of hypnosis, dance, music, and art therapy, as well as prayer and mental healing.

Biological-Based Therapies

This category of CAM includes natural and biological-based practices, interventions, and products, many of which overlap with conventional medicine's use of dietary supplements. This category includes herbal, special dietary, orthomolecular, and individual biological therapies.

Herbal therapy employs an individual herb or a mixture of herbs for healing purposes. An herb is a plant or plant part that produces and contains chemical substances that act upon the body. Special diet therapies, such as those proposed by Drs. Atkins, Ornish, Pritikin, and Weil, are believed to prevent and/or control illness as well as promote health. Orthomolecular therapies aim to treat disease with varying concentrations of chemicals such as magnesium, melatonin, and mega-doses of vitamins. Biological therapies include, for example, the use of laetrile and shark cartilage to treat cancer and the use of bee pollen to treat autoimmune and inflammatory diseases.

Manipulative and Body-Based Methods

This category includes methods that are based on manipulation and/or movement of the body. For example, chiropractors focus on the relationship between structure and function, primarily pertaining to the spine, and how that relationship affects the preservation and restoration of health. Chiropractors use manipulative therapy as an integral treatment tool.

In contrast, osteopaths place particular emphasis on the musculoskeletal system and practice osteopathic manipulation. Osteopaths believe that all of the body's systems work together and that disturbances in one system may have an impact upon function elsewhere in the body. Massage therapists manipulate the soft tissues of the body to normalize those tissues.

Energy Therapies

Energy therapies focus on energy fields originating within the body (biofields) or those from other sources (electromagnetic fields). Biofield therapies are intended to affect energy fields (the existence of which is not yet experimentally proven) that surround and penetrate the human body. Some forms of energy therapy manipulate biofields by applying pressure and/or manipulating the body by placing the hands in or through these fields. Examples include Qi gong, Reiki and Therapeutic Touch.

Qi gong is a component of traditional oriental medicine that combines movement, meditation, and regulation of breathing to enhance the flow of vital energy (qi) in the body, improve blood circulation, and enhance immune function. Reiki, the Japanese word representing Universal Life Energy, is based on the belief that, by channeling spiritual energy through the practitioner, the spirit is healed and, in turn, heals the physical body. Therapeutic Touch is derived from the ancient technique of "laying-on of hands." It is based on the premises that the therapist's healing force affects the patient's recovery and that healing is promoted when the body's energies are in balance. By passing their hands over the patient, these healers identify energy imbalances.

Bioelectromagnetic-based therapies involve the unconventional use of electromagnetic fields to treat illnesses or manage pain. These therapies are often used to treat asthma, cancer, and migraine headaches. Types of electromagnetic fields which are manipulated in these therapies include pulsed fields, magnetic fields, and alternating current or direct current fields.

Can Alternatives Affect My Treatment?

A critical issue in pursuing complementary alternatives mentioned thus far is the risk that these might have undesirable interactions with your medical treatment. It becomes all the more important to speak with your doctor who can offer advice on the use of alternatives. Official sources confirm this view. Though written for women, we find that the National Women's Health Information Center's advice on pursuing alternative medicine is appropriate for patients of both genders and all ages.[44]

---

[44] Adapted from **http://www.4woman.gov/faq/alternative.htm** .

Is It Okay to Want Both Traditional and Alternative Medicine?

Should you wish to explore non-traditional types of treatment, be sure to discuss all issues concerning treatments and therapies with your healthcare provider, whether a physician or practitioner of complementary and alternative medicine. Competent healthcare management requires knowledge of both conventional and alternative therapies you are taking for the practitioner to have a complete picture of your treatment plan.

The decision to use complementary and alternative treatments is an important one. Consider before selecting an alternative therapy, the safety and effectiveness of the therapy or treatment, the expertise and qualifications of the healthcare practitioner, and the quality of delivery. These topics should be considered when selecting any practitioner or therapy.

Finding CAM References on Vitiligo

Having read the previous discussion, you may be wondering which complementary or alternative treatments might be appropriate for vitiligo. For the remainder of this chapter, we will direct you to a number of official sources which can assist you in researching studies and publications. Some of these articles are rather technical, so some patience may be required.

National Center for Complementary and Alternative Medicine

The National Center for Complementary and Alternative Medicine (NCCAM) of the National Institutes of Health (http://nccam.nih.gov) has created a link to the National Library of Medicine's databases to allow patients to search for articles that specifically relate to vitiligo and complementary medicine. To search the database, go to the following Web site: **www.nlm.nih.gov/nccam/camonpubmed.html**. Select "CAM on PubMed." Enter "vitiligo" (or synonyms) into the search box. Click "Go." The following references provide information on particular aspects of complementary and alternative medicine (CAM) that are related to vitiligo:

- **Abnormalities of the auditory brainstem response in vitiligo.**
  Author(s): Nikiforidis GC, Tsambaos DG, Karamitsos DS, Koutsojannis CC, Georgiou SV.
  Source: Scand Audiol. 1993; 22(2): 97-100.
  http://www.ncbi.nlm.nih.gov:80/entrez/query.fcgi?cmd=Retrieve&db=PubMed&list_uids=8322003&dopt=Abstract

- **Atypical Kaposi's sarcoma in a patient with vitiligo and pernicious anemia.**
  Author(s): Ruzicka T.
  Source: Dermatologica. 1981; 163(2): 199-204. No Abstract Available.
  http://www.ncbi.nlm.nih.gov:80/entrez/query.fcgi?cmd=Retrieve&db=
  PubMed&list_uids=7286359&dopt=Abstract

- **Childhood vitiligo successfully treated with bath PUVA.**
  Author(s): Mai DW, Omohundro C, Dijkstra JW, Bailin PL.
  Source: Pediatr Dermatol. 1998 January-February; 15(1): 53-5.
  http://www.ncbi.nlm.nih.gov:80/entrez/query.fcgi?cmd=Retrieve&db=
  PubMed&list_uids=9496807&dopt=Abstract

- **Current treatment of vitiligo in China.**
  Author(s): Shao C, Ye G.
  Source: Chin Med J (Engl). 1995 September; 108(9): 647-9. Review. No
  Abstract Available.
  http://www.ncbi.nlm.nih.gov:80/entrez/query.fcgi?cmd=Retrieve&db=
  PubMed&list_uids=8575227&dopt=Abstract

- **Historic view of vitiligo in Korea.**
  Author(s): Hann SK, Chung HS.
  Source: Int J Dermatol. 1997 April; 36(4): 313-5. No Abstract Available.
  http://www.ncbi.nlm.nih.gov:80/entrez/query.fcgi?cmd=Retrieve&db=
  PubMed&list_uids=9169339&dopt=Abstract

- **Improvement of vitiligo after oral treatment with vitamin B12 and folic acid and the importance of sun exposure.**
  Author(s): Juhlin L, Olsson MJ.
  Source: Acta Derm Venereol. 1997 November; 77(6): 460-2.
  http://www.ncbi.nlm.nih.gov:80/entrez/query.fcgi?cmd=Retrieve&db=
  PubMed&list_uids=9394983&dopt=Abstract

- **In vitro assessment of 'T' lymphocyte functioning in vitiligo. Support for autoimmune hypothesis concerning the disease.**
  Author(s): Taher-Uz-Zaman, Begum S, Waheed MA.
  Source: Acta Derm Venereol. 1992 August; 72(4): 266-7.
  http://www.ncbi.nlm.nih.gov:80/entrez/query.fcgi?cmd=Retrieve&db=
  PubMed&list_uids=1357881&dopt=Abstract

- **In vivo and in vitro evidence for hydrogen peroxide (H2O2) accumulation in the epidermis of patients with vitiligo and its**

successful removal by a UVB-activated pseudocatalase.
Author(s): Schallreuter KU, Moore J, Wood JM, Beazley WD, Gaze DC, Tobin DJ, Marshall HS, Panske A, Panzig E, Hibberts NA.
Source: J Investig Dermatol Symp Proc. 1999 September; 4(1): 91-6. Review.
http://www.ncbi.nlm.nih.gov:80/entrez/query.fcgi?cmd=Retrieve&db=PubMed&list_uids=10537016&dopt=Abstract

- **Investigation of the effect of Angelica sinensis root extract on the proliferation of melanocytes in culture.**
  Author(s): Raman A, Lin ZX, Sviderskaya E, Kowalska D.
  Source: J Ethnopharmacol. 1996 November; 54(2-3): 165-70.
  http://www.ncbi.nlm.nih.gov:80/entrez/query.fcgi?cmd=Retrieve&db=PubMed&list_uids=8953431&dopt=Abstract

- **Letter: Vitiligo in ancient Indian medicine.**
  Author(s): Singh G, Ansari Z, Dwivedi RN.
  Source: Arch Dermatol. 1974 June; 109(6): 913. No Abstract Available.
  http://www.ncbi.nlm.nih.gov:80/entrez/query.fcgi?cmd=Retrieve&db=PubMed&list_uids=4598079&dopt=Abstract

- **Management of vitiligo.**
  Author(s): Nordlund JJ, Halder RM, Grimes P.
  Source: Dermatol Clin. 1993 January; 11(1): 27-33.
  http://www.ncbi.nlm.nih.gov:80/entrez/query.fcgi?cmd=Retrieve&db=PubMed&list_uids=8435915&dopt=Abstract

- **Picrorhiza kurroa, an ayurvedic herb, may potentiate photochemotherapy in vitiligo.**
  Author(s): Bedi KL, Zutshi U, Chopra CL, Amla V.
  Source: J Ethnopharmacol. 1989 December; 27(3): 347-52. No Abstract Available.
  http://www.ncbi.nlm.nih.gov:80/entrez/query.fcgi?cmd=Retrieve&db=PubMed&list_uids=2615440&dopt=Abstract

- **Psoralen photochemotherapy.**
  Author(s): Gupta AK, Anderson TF.
  Source: J Am Acad Dermatol. 1987 November; 17(5 Pt 1): 703-34. Review.
  http://www.ncbi.nlm.nih.gov:80/entrez/query.fcgi?cmd=Retrieve&db=PubMed&list_uids=3316316&dopt=Abstract

- **Retrospective ocular study of patients receiving oral 8-methoxypsoralen and solar irradiation for the treatment of vitiligo.**
  Author(s): El-Mofty AM, El-Mofty A.
  Source: Ann Ophthalmol. 1979 June; 11(6): 946-8.
  http://www.ncbi.nlm.nih.gov:80/entrez/query.fcgi?cmd=Retrieve&db=PubMed&list_uids=496187&dopt=Abstract

- **Sulphorhodamine B assay for measuring proliferation of a pigmented melanocyte cell line and its application to the evaluation of crude drugs used in the treatment of vitiligo.**
  Author(s): Lin ZX, Hoult JR, Raman A.
  Source: J Ethnopharmacol. 1999 August; 66(2): 141-50.
  http://www.ncbi.nlm.nih.gov:80/entrez/query.fcgi?cmd=Retrieve&db=PubMed&list_uids=10433470&dopt=Abstract

- **Treatment of vitiligo based on the principle of pacifying liver by resolving stasis and activating blood circulation, plus exorcising "wind". An observation on therapeutic effects in 100 cases.**
  Author(s): Zhu GD.
  Source: J Tradit Chin Med. 1982 March; 2(1): 71-5. No Abstract Available.
  http://www.ncbi.nlm.nih.gov:80/entrez/query.fcgi?cmd=Retrieve&db=PubMed&list_uids=6765693&dopt=Abstract

- **Vitiligo--a retrospect.**
  Author(s): Nair BK.
  Source: Int J Dermatol. 1978 November; 17(9): 755-7. No Abstract Available.
  http://www.ncbi.nlm.nih.gov:80/entrez/query.fcgi?cmd=Retrieve&db=PubMed&list_uids=365814&dopt=Abstract

- **Vitiligo-like leucoderma during photochemotherapy for mycosis fungoides.**
  Author(s): Mimouni D, David M, Feinmesser M, Coire C I, Hodak E.
  Source: Br J Dermatol. 2001 December; 145(6): 1008-14.
  http://www.ncbi.nlm.nih.gov:80/entrez/query.fcgi?cmd=Retrieve&db=PubMed&list_uids=11899124&dopt=Abstract

Additional Web Resources

A number of additional Web sites offer encyclopedic information covering CAM and related topics. The following is a representative sample:

- Alternative Medicine Foundation, Inc.: **http://www.herbmed.org/**

- AOL: **http://search.aol.com/cat.adp?id=169&layer=&from=subcats**

- Chinese Medicine: **http://www.newcenturynutrition.com/**

- drkoop.com®: **http://www.drkoop.com/InteractiveMedicine/IndexC.html**

- Family Village: **http://www.familyvillage.wisc.edu/med_altn.htm**

- Google: **http://directory.google.com/Top/Health/Alternative/**

- Healthnotes: **http://www.thedacare.org/healthnotes/**

- Open Directory Project: **http://dmoz.org/Health/Alternative/**

- TPN.com: **http://www.tnp.com/**

- Yahoo.com: **http://dir.yahoo.com/Health/Alternative_Medicine/**

- WebMD®Health: **http://my.webmd.com/drugs_and_herbs**

- WellNet: **http://www.wellnet.ca/herbsa-c.htm**

- WholeHealthMD.com: **http://www.wholehealthmd.com/reflib/0,1529,,00.html**

The following is a specific Web list relating to vitiligo; please note that any particular subject below may indicate either a therapeutic use, or a contraindication (potential danger), and does not reflect an official recommendation:

- **General Overview**

  Vitiligo
  Source: Healthnotes, Inc.; www.healthnotes.com
  Hyperlink:
  http://www.thedacare.org/healthnotes/Concern/Vitiligo.htm

  Vitiligo
  Source: Integrative Medicine Communications; www.onemedicine.com

Hyperlink:
http://www.drkoop.com/InteractiveMedicine/ConsLookups/Uses/viti
ligo.html

- **Chinese Medicine**

  Gusuibu
  Alternative names: Fortune's Drynaria Rhizome; Rhizoma Drynariae
  Source: Chinese Materia Medica
  Hyperlink: http://www.newcenturynutrition.com/

  Tusizi
  Alternative names: Dodder Seed; Semen Cuseutae
  Source: Chinese Materia Medica
  Hyperlink: http://www.newcenturynutrition.com/

- **Herbs and Supplements**

  Amino Acids Overview
  Source: Healthnotes, Inc.; www.healthnotes.com
  Hyperlink:
  http://www.thedacare.org/healthnotes/Supp/Amino_Acids.htm

  L-Phenylalanine
  Source: Healthnotes, Inc.; www.healthnotes.com
  Hyperlink:
  http://www.thedacare.org/healthnotes/Concern/Vitiligo.htm

  PABA
  Source: Healthnotes, Inc.; www.healthnotes.com
  Hyperlink: http://www.thedacare.org/healthnotes/Supp/PABA.htm

  PABA
  Source: Healthnotes, Inc.; www.healthnotes.com
  Hyperlink:
  http://www.thedacare.org/healthnotes/Concern/Vitiligo.htm

  PABA
  Source: WholeHealthMD.com, LLC.; www.wholehealthmd.com
  Hyperlink:
  http://www.wholehealthmd.com/refshelf/substances_view/0,1525,100
  49,00.html

PABA (Para-Aminobenzoic Acid)
Source: Prima Communications, Inc.
Hyperlink: http://www.personalhealthzone.com/pg000217.html

Phenylalanine
Source: Healthnotes, Inc.; www.healthnotes.com
Hyperlink:
http://www.thedacare.org/healthnotes/Supp/Phenylalanine.htm

Phenylalanine
Source: Healthnotes, Inc.; www.healthnotes.com
Hyperlink:
http://www.thedacare.org/healthnotes/Concern/Vitiligo.htm

Phenylalanine
Source: Integrative Medicine Communications; www.onemedicine.com
Hyperlink:
http://www.drkoop.com/interactivemedicine/ConsSupplements/Phen
ylalaninecs.html

Phenylalanine
Source: Prima Communications, Inc.
Hyperlink: http://www.personalhealthzone.com/pg000141.html

Picrorhiza
Source: Healthnotes, Inc.; www.healthnotes.com
Hyperlink:
http://www.thedacare.org/healthnotes/Concern/Vitiligo.htm

Picrorhiza
Alternative names: Picrorhiza kurroa
Source: Healthnotes, Inc.; www.healthnotes.com
Hyperlink:
http://www.thedacare.org/healthnotes/Herb/Picrorhiza.htm

- **Related Conditions**

Indigestion, Heartburn, and Low Stomach Acidity
Source: Healthnotes, Inc.; www.healthnotes.com
Hyperlink:
http://www.thedacare.org/healthnotes/Concern/Indigestion.htm

General References

A good place to find general background information on CAM is the National Library of Medicine. It has prepared within the MEDLINEplus system an information topic page dedicated to complementary and alternative medicine. To access this page, go to the MEDLINEplus site at: **www.nlm.nih.gov/medlineplus/alternativemedicine.html.** This Web site provides a general overview of various topics and can lead to a number of general sources. The following additional references describe, in broad terms, alternative and complementary medicine (sorted alphabetically by title; hyperlinks provide rankings, information, and reviews at Amazon.com):

- **The Skin Cancer Answer** by I. William Lane, et al; Paperback - 160 pages (February 1999), Avery Penguin Putnam; ISBN: 0895298651; http://www.amazon.com/exec/obidos/ASIN/0895298651/icongroupinterna

- **Smart Medicine for Your Skin: A Comprehensive Guide to Understanding Conventional and Alternative Therapies to Heal Common Skin Problems** by Jeanette Jacknin, M.D.; Paperback - 414 pages (August 6, 2001), Avery Penguin Putnam; ISBN: 1583330984; http://www.amazon.com/exec/obidos/ASIN/1583330984/icongroupinterna

- **Alternative Medicine for Dummies** by James Dillard (Author); Audio Cassette, Abridged edition (1998), Harper Audio; ISBN: 0694520659; http://www.amazon.com/exec/obidos/ASIN/0694520659/icongroupinterna

- **Complementary and Alternative Medicine Secrets** by W. Kohatsu (Editor); Hardcover (2001), Hanley & Belfus; ISBN: 1560534400; http://www.amazon.com/exec/obidos/ASIN/1560534400/icongroupinterna

- **Dictionary of Alternative Medicine** by J. C. Segen; Paperback-2nd edition (2001), Appleton & Lange; ISBN: 0838516211; http://www.amazon.com/exec/obidos/ASIN/0838516211/icongroupinterna

- **Eat, Drink, and Be Healthy: The Harvard Medical School Guide to Healthy Eating** by Walter C. Willett, MD, et al; Hardcover - 352 pages (2001), Simon & Schuster; ISBN: 0684863375; http://www.amazon.com/exec/obidos/ASIN/0684863375/icongroupinterna

- **Encyclopedia of Natural Medicine, Revised 2nd Edition** by Michael T. Murray, Joseph E. Pizzorno; Paperback - 960 pages, 2nd Rev edition (1997), Prima Publishing; ISBN: 0761511571; http://www.amazon.com/exec/obidos/ASIN/0761511571/icongroupinterna

- **Integrative Medicine: An Introduction to the Art & Science of Healing** by Andrew Weil (Author); Audio Cassette, Unabridged edition (2001), Sounds

True; ISBN: 1564558541;
http://www.amazon.com/exec/obidos/ASIN/1564558541/icongroupinterna

- **New Encyclopedia of Herbs & Their Uses** by Deni Bown; Hardcover - 448 pages, Revised edition (2001), DK Publishing; ISBN: 078948031X; http://www.amazon.com/exec/obidos/ASIN/078948031X/icongroupinterna

- **Textbook of Complementary and Alternative Medicine** by Wayne B. Jonas; Hardcover (2003), Lippincott, Williams & Wilkins; ISBN: 0683044370; http://www.amazon.com/exec/obidos/ASIN/0683044370/icongroupinterna

For additional information on complementary and alternative medicine, ask your doctor or write to:

National Institutes of Health
National Center for Complementary and Alternative Medicine Clearinghouse
P. O. Box 8218
Silver Spring, MD 20907-8218

Vocabulary Builder

The following vocabulary builder gives definitions of words used in this chapter that have not been defined in previous chapters:

Alkaloid: One of a large group of nitrogenous basis substances found in plants. They are usually very bitter and many are pharmacologically active. Examples are atropine, caffeine, coniine, morphine, nicotine, quinine, strychnine. The term is also applied to synthetic substances (artificial a's) which have structures similar to plant alkaloids, such as procaine. [EU]

Papillomavirus: A genus of papovaviridae causing proliferation of the epithelium, which may lead to malignancy. A wide range of animals are infected including humans, chimpanzees, cattle, rabbits, dogs, and horses. [NIH]

Percutaneous: Performed through the skin, as injection of radiopacque material in radiological examination, or the removal of tissue for biopsy accomplished by a needle. [EU]

Psychiatry: The medical science that deals with the origin, diagnosis, prevention, and treatment of mental disorders. [NIH]

APPENDIX C. RESEARCHING NUTRITION

Overview

Since the time of Hippocrates, doctors have understood the importance of diet and nutrition to patients' health and well-being. Since then, they have accumulated an impressive archive of studies and knowledge dedicated to this subject. Based on their experience, doctors and healthcare providers may recommend particular dietary supplements to patients with vitiligo. Any dietary recommendation is based on a patient's age, body mass, gender, lifestyle, eating habits, food preferences, and health condition. It is therefore likely that different patients with vitiligo may be given different recommendations. Some recommendations may be directly related to vitiligo, while others may be more related to the patient's general health. These recommendations, themselves, may differ from what official sources recommend for the average person.

In this chapter we will begin by briefly reviewing the essentials of diet and nutrition that will broadly frame more detailed discussions of vitiligo. We will then show you how to find studies dedicated specifically to nutrition and vitiligo.

Food and Nutrition: General Principles

What Are Essential Foods?

Food is generally viewed by official sources as consisting of six basic elements: (1) fluids, (2) carbohydrates, (3) protein, (4) fats, (5) vitamins, and (6) minerals. Consuming a combination of these elements is considered to be a healthy diet:

- **Fluids** are essential to human life as 80-percent of the body is composed of water. Water is lost via urination, sweating, diarrhea, vomiting, diuretics (drugs that increase urination), caffeine, and physical exertion.

- **Carbohydrates** are the main source for human energy (thermoregulation) and the bulk of typical diets. They are mostly classified as being either simple or complex. Simple carbohydrates include sugars which are often consumed in the form of cookies, candies, or cakes. Complex carbohydrates consist of starches and dietary fibers. Starches are consumed in the form of pastas, breads, potatoes, rice, and other foods. Soluble fibers can be eaten in the form of certain vegetables, fruits, oats, and legumes. Insoluble fibers include brown rice, whole grains, certain fruits, wheat bran and legumes.

- **Proteins** are eaten to build and repair human tissues. Some foods that are high in protein are also high in fat and calories. Food sources for protein include nuts, meat, fish, cheese, and other dairy products.

- **Fats** are consumed for both energy and the absorption of certain vitamins. There are many types of fats, with many general publications recommending the intake of unsaturated fats or those low in cholesterol.

Vitamins and minerals are fundamental to human health, growth, and, in some cases, disease prevention. Most are consumed in your diet (exceptions being vitamins K and D which are produced by intestinal bacteria and sunlight on the skin, respectively). Each vitamin and mineral plays a different role in health. The following outlines essential vitamins:

- **Vitamin A** is important to the health of your eyes, hair, bones, and skin; sources of vitamin A include foods such as eggs, carrots, and cantaloupe.

- **Vitamin B1**, also known as thiamine, is important for your nervous system and energy production; food sources for thiamine include meat, peas, fortified cereals, bread, and whole grains.

- **Vitamin B2**, also known as riboflavin, is important for your nervous system and muscles, but is also involved in the release of proteins from nutrients; food sources for riboflavin include dairy products, leafy vegetables, meat, and eggs.

- **Vitamin B^3**, also known as niacin, is important for healthy skin and helps the body use energy; food sources for niacin include peas, peanuts, fish, and whole grains

- **Vitamin B^6**, also known as pyridoxine, is important for the regulation of cells in the nervous system and is vital for blood formation; food sources for pyridoxine include bananas, whole grains, meat, and fish.

- **Vitamin B^{12}** is vital for a healthy nervous system and for the growth of red blood cells in bone marrow; food sources for vitamin B^{12} include yeast, milk, fish, eggs, and meat.

- **Vitamin C** allows the body's immune system to fight various diseases, strengthens body tissue, and improves the body's use of iron; food sources for vitamin C include a wide variety of fruits and vegetables.

- **Vitamin D** helps the body absorb calcium which strengthens bones and teeth; food sources for vitamin D include oily fish and dairy products.

- **Vitamin E** can help protect certain organs and tissues from various degenerative diseases; food sources for vitamin E include margarine, vegetables, eggs, and fish.

- **Vitamin K** is essential for bone formation and blood clotting; common food sources for vitamin K include leafy green vegetables.

- **Folic Acid** maintains healthy cells and blood and, when taken by a pregnant woman, can prevent her fetus from developing neural tube defects; food sources for folic acid include nuts, fortified breads, leafy green vegetables, and whole grains.

It should be noted that one can overdose on certain vitamins which become toxic if consumed in excess (e.g. vitamin A, D, E and K).

Like vitamins, minerals are chemicals that are required by the body to remain in good health. Because the human body does not manufacture these chemicals internally, we obtain them from food and other dietary sources. The more important minerals include:

- **Calcium** is needed for healthy bones, teeth, and muscles, but also helps the nervous system function; food sources for calcium include dry beans, peas, eggs, and dairy products.

- **Chromium** is helpful in regulating sugar levels in blood; food sources for chromium include egg yolks, raw sugar, cheese, nuts, beets, whole grains, and meat.

- **Fluoride** is used by the body to help prevent tooth decay and to reinforce bone strength; sources of fluoride include drinking water and certain brands of toothpaste.

- **Iodine** helps regulate the body's use of energy by synthesizing into the hormone thyroxine; food sources include leafy green vegetables, nuts, egg yolks, and red meat.

- **Iron** helps maintain muscles and the formation of red blood cells and certain proteins; food sources for iron include meat, dairy products, eggs, and leafy green vegetables.

- **Magnesium** is important for the production of DNA, as well as for healthy teeth, bones, muscles, and nerves; food sources for magnesium include dried fruit, dark green vegetables, nuts, and seafood.

- **Phosphorous** is used by the body to work with calcium to form bones and teeth; food sources for phosphorous include eggs, meat, cereals, and dairy products.

- **Selenium** primarily helps maintain normal heart and liver functions; food sources for selenium include wholegrain cereals, fish, meat, and dairy products.

- **Zinc** helps wounds heal, the formation of sperm, and encourage rapid growth and energy; food sources include dried beans, shellfish, eggs, and nuts.

The United States government periodically publishes recommended diets and consumption levels of the various elements of food. Again, your doctor may encourage deviations from the average official recommendation based on your specific condition. To learn more about basic dietary guidelines, visit the Web site: **http://www.health.gov/dietaryguidelines/**. Based on these guidelines, many foods are required to list the nutrition levels on the food's packaging. Labeling Requirements are listed at the following site maintained by the Food and Drug Administration: **http://www.cfsan.fda.gov/~dms/lab-cons.html**. When interpreting these requirements, the government recommends that consumers become familiar with the following abbreviations before reading FDA literature:[45]

- **DVs (Daily Values):** A new dietary reference term that will appear on the food label. It is made up of two sets of references, DRVs and RDIs.

- **DRVs (Daily Reference Values):** A set of dietary references that applies to fat, saturated fat, cholesterol, carbohydrate, protein, fiber, sodium, and potassium.

---

[45] Adapted from the FDA: **http://www.fda.gov/fdac/special/foodlabel/dvs.html**.

- **RDIs (Reference Daily Intakes):** A set of dietary references based on the Recommended Dietary Allowances for essential vitamins and minerals and, in selected groups, protein. The name "RDI" replaces the term "U.S. RDA."

- **RDAs (Recommended Dietary Allowances):** A set of estimated nutrient allowances established by the National Academy of Sciences. It is updated periodically to reflect current scientific knowledge.

What Are Dietary Supplements?[46]

Dietary supplements are widely available through many commercial sources, including health food stores, grocery stores, pharmacies, and by mail. Dietary supplements are provided in many forms including tablets, capsules, powders, gel-tabs, extracts, and liquids. Historically in the United States, the most prevalent type of dietary supplement was a multivitamin/mineral tablet or capsule that was available in pharmacies, either by prescription or "over the counter." Supplements containing strictly herbal preparations were less widely available. Currently in the United States, a wide array of supplement products are available, including vitamin, mineral, other nutrients, and botanical supplements as well as ingredients and extracts of animal and plant origin.

The Office of Dietary Supplements (ODS) of the National Institutes of Health is the official agency of the United States which has the expressed goal of acquiring "new knowledge to help prevent, detect, diagnose, and treat disease and disability, from the rarest genetic disorder to the common cold."[47] According to the ODS, dietary supplements can have an important impact on the prevention and management of disease and on the maintenance of health.[48] The ODS notes that considerable research on the effects of dietary supplements has been conducted in Asia and Europe where the use of plant products, in particular, has a long tradition. However, the

---

[46] This discussion has been adapted from the NIH: http://ods.od.nih.gov/whatare/whatare.html.

[47] Contact: The Office of Dietary Supplements, National Institutes of Health, Building 31, Room 1B29, 31 Center Drive, MSC 2086, Bethesda, Maryland 20892-2086, Tel: (301) 435-2920, Fax: (301) 480-1845, E-mail: **ods@nih.gov**.

[48] Adapted from **http://ods.od.nih.gov/about/about.html**. The Dietary Supplement Health and Education Act defines dietary supplements as "a product (other than tobacco) intended to supplement the diet that bears or contains one or more of the following dietary ingredients: a vitamin, mineral, amino acid, herb or other botanical; or a dietary substance for use to supplement the diet by increasing the total dietary intake; or a concentrate, metabolite, constituent, extract, or combination of any ingredient described above; and intended for ingestion in the form of a capsule, powder, softgel, or gelcap, and not represented as a conventional food or as a sole item of a meal or the diet."

overwhelming majority of supplements have not been studied scientifically. To explore the role of dietary supplements in the improvement of health care, the ODS plans, organizes, and supports conferences, workshops, and symposia on scientific topics related to dietary supplements. The ODS often works in conjunction with other NIH Institutes and Centers, other government agencies, professional organizations, and public advocacy groups.

To learn more about official information on dietary supplements, visit the ODS site at **http://ods.od.nih.gov/whatare/whatare.html**. Or contact:

> The Office of Dietary Supplements
> National Institutes of Health
> Building 31, Room 1B29
> 31 Center Drive, MSC 2086
> Bethesda, Maryland 20892-2086
> Tel: (301) 435-2920
> Fax: (301) 480-1845
> E-mail: ods@nih.gov

Finding Studies on Vitiligo

The NIH maintains an office dedicated to patient nutrition and diet. The National Institutes of Health's Office of Dietary Supplements (ODS) offers a searchable bibliographic database called the IBIDS (International Bibliographic Information on Dietary Supplements). The IBIDS contains over 460,000 scientific citations and summaries about dietary supplements and nutrition as well as references to published international, scientific literature on dietary supplements such as vitamins, minerals, and botanicals.[49] IBIDS is available to the public free of charge through the ODS Internet page: **http://ods.od.nih.gov/databases/ibids.html**.

After entering the search area, you have three choices: (1) IBIDS Consumer Database, (2) Full IBIDS Database, or (3) Peer Reviewed Citations Only. We recommend that you start with the Consumer Database. While you may not find references for the topics that are of most interest to you, check back periodically as this database is frequently updated. More studies can be

---

[49] Adapted from http://ods.od.nih.gov. IBIDS is produced by the Office of Dietary Supplements (ODS) at the National Institutes of Health to assist the public, healthcare providers, educators, and researchers in locating credible, scientific information on dietary supplements. IBIDS was developed and will be maintained through an interagency partnership with the Food and Nutrition Information Center of the National Agricultural Library, U.S. Department of Agriculture.

found by searching the Full IBIDS Database. Healthcare professionals and researchers generally use the third option, which lists peer-reviewed citations. In all cases, we suggest that you take advantage of the "Advanced Search" option that allows you to retrieve up to 100 fully explained references in a comprehensive format. Type "vitiligo" (or synonyms) into the search box. To narrow the search, you can also select the "Title" field.

The following information is typical of that found when using the "Full IBIDS Database" when searching using "vitiligo" (or a synonym):

- **Alterations in IL-6, IL-8, GM-CSF, TNF-alpha, and IFN-gamma release by peripheral mononuclear cells in patients with active vitiligo.**
  Author(s): Department of Dermatology, Kaohsiung Medical College, Taiwan.
  Source: Yu, H S Chang, K L Yu, C L Li, H F Wu, M T Wu, C S Wu, C S J-Invest-Dermatol. 1997 April; 108(4): 527-9 0022-202X

- **Analysis of esterification of retinoids in the retinal pigmented epithelium of the Mitf-vit (vitiligo) mutant mouse.**
  Author(s): Department of Cellular Biology and Anatomy, Medical College of Georgia, Augusta, Georgia 30912-2000, USA.
  Source: Evans, B L Smith, S B Mol-Vis. 1997 October 24; 311 1090-0535

- **Antioxidant status in the blood of patients with active vitiligo.**
  Author(s): San Gallicano Dermatological Institute, Rome, Italy.
  Source: Picardo, M Passi, S Morrone, A Grandinetti, M Di Carlo, A Ippolito, F Pigment-Cell-Res. 1994 April; 7(2): 110-5 0893-5785

- **Calcipotriol in vitiligo: a preliminary study.**
  Author(s): Department of Dermatology, Himalayan Institute of Medical Sciences, Jolly Grant, Dehradun, India. dprsaini@nde.vsnl.net.in
  Source: Parsad, D Saini, R Nagpal, R Pediatr-Dermatol. 1999 Jul-August; 16(4): 317-20 0736-8046

- **Chronic arsenicism with vitiligo, hyperthyroidism, and cancer.**
  Source: Bickley, L K Papa, C M N-J-Med. 1989 May; 86(5): 377-80 0885-842X

- **Combination of clobetasol and tretinoin in vitiligo -letter-.**
  Source: Parsad, D Saini, R Juneja, A Int-J-Dermatol. 2000 August; 39(8): 639-40 0011-9059

- **Combination of PUVAsol and topical calcipotriol in vitiligo.**
  Author(s): Department of Dermatology, HIMS, Dehradun, India.
  Source: Parsad, D Saini, R Verma, N Dermatology. 1998; 197(2): 167-70 1018-8665

- **Current treatment of vitiligo in China.**
  Author(s): Institute of Dermatology, Chinese Academy of Medical Sciences, Nanjing.
  Source: Shao, C Ye, G Chin-Med-J-(Engl). 1995 September; 108(9): 647-9 0366-6999

- **Delayed rhodopsin regeneration and altered distribution of interphotoreceptor retinoid binding protein (IRBP) in the mi(vit)/mi(vit) (vitiligo) mouse.**
  Author(s): Department of Cellular Biology and Anatomy, Medical College of Georgia, Augusta, USA.
  Source: Smith, S B McClung, J Wiggert, B N Nir, I J-Neurocytol. 1997 September; 26(9): 605-13 0300-4864

- **Depigmentation therapy in vitiligo universalis with topical 4-methoxyphenol and the Q-switched ruby laser.**
  Author(s): Netherlands Institute for Pigmentary Disorders, Amsterdam.
  Source: Njoo, M D Vodegel, R M Westerhof, W J-Am-Acad-Dermatol. 2000 May; 42(5 Pt 1): 760-9 0190-9622

- **Depigmentation therapy with Q-switched ruby laser after tanning in vitiligo universalis.**
  Author(s): Department of Dermatology, Chosun University Hospital, Gwangju, Korea. yjkim@mail.chosun.ac.kr
  Source: Kim, Y J Chung, B S Choi, K C Dermatol-Surg. 2001 November; 27(11): 969-70 1076-0512

- **Discussion of a case of vitiligo.**
  Author(s): Department of Dermatology, University of Texas Southwestern Medical Center, Dallas 75235, USA.
  Source: Lerner, M R Fitzpatrick, T B Halder, R M Hawk, J L Photodermatol-Photoimmunol-Photomed. 1999 February; 15(1): 41-4 0905-4383

- **Dopa responsive dystonia in a girl with vitiligo.**
  Author(s): Department of Neurology, K.E.M. Hospital, Parel, Mumbai, India.
  Source: Chaudhary, N Mani, J Rawat, S Mulye, R Shah, P Indian-Pediatr. 1998 July; 35(7): 663-5 0019-6061

- **Epidermal oxidative stress in vitiligo.**
  Author(s): Centro Invecchiamento Cellulare, Istituto Dermopatico dell'Immacolata (IRCCS), Roma, Italy.
  Source: Passi, S Grandinetti, M Maggio, F Stancato, A De Luca, C Pigment-Cell-Res. 1998 April; 11(2): 81-5 0893-5785

- **Experience with calcipotriol as adjunctive treatment for vitiligo in patients who do not respond to PUVA alone: a preliminary study.**
  Author(s): Department of Dermatology, Hacettepe University School of Medicine, Ankara, Turkey.
  Source: Yalcin, B Sahin, S Bukulmez, G Karaduman, A Atakan, N Akan, T Kolemen, F J-Am-Acad-Dermatol. 2001 April; 44(4): 634-7 0190-9622

- **Folic acid and vitamin B12 in vitiligo: a nutritional approach.**
  Author(s): Department of Dermatology, University of Alabama, Birmingham Medical Center.
  Source: Montes, L F Diaz, M L Lajous, J Garcia, N J Cutis. 1992 July; 50(1): 39-42 0011-4162

- **Guidelines for the treatment of vitiligo.**
  Author(s): University of Athens, School of Medicine, Department of Dermatology, Greece.
  Source: Antoniou, C Katsambas, A Drugs. 1992 April; 43(4): 490-8 0012-6667

- **Historic view of vitiligo in Korea.**
  Author(s): Department of Dermatology, Yonsei University College of Medicine, Seoul, Korea.
  Source: Hann, S K Chung, H S Int-J-Dermatol. 1997 April; 36(4): 313-5 0011-9059

- **Identification of pigment cell antigens defined by vitiligo antibodies.**
  Author(s): Department of Dermatology, New York University School of Medicine, NY 10016.
  Source: Cui, J Harning, R Henn, M Bystryn, J C J-Invest-Dermatol. 1992 February; 98(2): 162-5 0022-202X

- **Immunohistochemical study of ACTH and alpha-MSH in vitiligo patients successfully treated with a sex steroid-thyroid hormone mixture.**
  Author(s): Department of Dermatology, Yamaguchi University School of Medicine, Ube, Japan.
  Source: Ichimiya, M J-Dermatol. 1999 August; 26(8): 502-6 0385-2407

Federal Resources on Nutrition

In addition to the IBIDS, the United States Department of Health and Human Services (HHS) and the United States Department of Agriculture (USDA) provide many sources of information on general nutrition and health. Recommended resources include:

- healthfinder®, HHS's gateway to health information, including diet and nutrition:
  http://www.healthfinder.gov/scripts/SearchContext.asp?topic=238&page=0

- The United States Department of Agriculture's Web site dedicated to nutrition information: **www.nutrition.gov**

- The Food and Drug Administration's Web site for federal food safety information: **www.foodsafety.gov**

- The National Action Plan on Overweight and Obesity sponsored by the United States Surgeon General:
  http://www.surgeongeneral.gov/topics/obesity/

- The Center for Food Safety and Applied Nutrition has an Internet site sponsored by the Food and Drug Administration and the Department of Health and Human Services: **http://vm.cfsan.fda.gov/**

- Center for Nutrition Policy and Promotion sponsored by the United States Department of Agriculture: **http://www.usda.gov/cnpp/**

- Food and Nutrition Information Center, National Agricultural Library sponsored by the United States Department of Agriculture: **http://www.nal.usda.gov/fnic/**

- Food and Nutrition Service sponsored by the United States Department of Agriculture: **http://www.fns.usda.gov/fns/**

Additional Web Resources

A number of additional Web sites offer encyclopedic information covering food and nutrition. The following is a representative sample:

- AOL: **http://search.aol.com/cat.adp?id=174&layer=&from=subcats**

- Family Village: **http://www.familyvillage.wisc.edu/med_nutrition.html**

- Google: **http://directory.google.com/Top/Health/Nutrition/**

- Healthnotes: **http://www.thedacare.org/healthnotes/**

- Open Directory Project: **http://dmoz.org/Health/Nutrition/**

- Yahoo.com: **http://dir.yahoo.com/Health/Nutrition/**

- WebMD®Health: **http://my.webmd.com/nutrition**

- WholeHealthMD.com:
  http://www.wholehealthmd.com/reflib/0,1529,,00.html

The following is a specific Web list relating to vitiligo; please note that any particular subject below may indicate either a therapeutic use, or a contraindication (potential danger), and does not reflect an official recommendation:

- **Vitamins**

  Folic Acid
  Source: Healthnotes, Inc.; www.healthnotes.com
  Hyperlink:
  http://www.thedacare.org/healthnotes/Supp/Folic_Acid.htm

  Vitamin B12
  Source: Healthnotes, Inc.; www.healthnotes.com
  Hyperlink:
  http://www.thedacare.org/healthnotes/Supp/Vitamin_B12.htm

  Vitamin C
  Source: Healthnotes, Inc.; www.healthnotes.com
  Hyperlink:
  http://www.thedacare.org/healthnotes/Supp/Vitamin_C.htm

  Vitamin D
  Source: Healthnotes, Inc.; www.healthnotes.com
  Hyperlink:
  http://www.thedacare.org/healthnotes/Supp/Vitamin_D.htm

- **Minerals**

  Betaine Hydrochloride
  Source: Healthnotes, Inc.; www.healthnotes.com
  Hyperlink:
  http://www.thedacare.org/healthnotes/Supp/Betaine_HCl.htm

Folate
Source: Prima Communications, Inc.
Hyperlink: http://www.personalhealthzone.com/pg000161.html

- **Food and Diet**

Cream
Source: Healthnotes, Inc.; www.healthnotes.com
Hyperlink:
http://www.thedacare.org/healthnotes/Concern/Vitiligo.htm

Vocabulary Builder

The following vocabulary builder defines words used in the references in this chapter that have not been defined in previous chapters:

ACTH: Adrenocorticotropic hormone. [EU]

Capsules: Hard or soft soluble containers used for the oral administration of medicine. [NIH]

Carbohydrate: An aldehyde or ketone derivative of a polyhydric alcohol, particularly of the pentahydric and hexahydric alcohols. They are so named because the hydrogen and oxygen are usually in the proportion to form water, (CH2O)n. The most important carbohydrates are the starches, sugars, celluloses, and gums. They are classified into mono-, di-, tri-, poly- and heterosaccharides. [EU]

Cholesterol: The principal sterol of all higher animals, distributed in body tissues, especially the brain and spinal cord, and in animal fats and oils. [NIH]

Clobetasol: Topical corticosteroid that is absorbed faster than fluocinonide. It is used in psoriasis, but may cause marked adrenocortical suppression. [NIH]

Diarrhea: Passage of excessively liquid or excessively frequent stools. [NIH]

Epithelium: The covering of internal and external surfaces of the body, including the lining of vessels and other small cavities. It consists of cells joined by small amounts of cementing substances. Epithelium is classified into types on the basis of the number of layers deep and the shape of the superficial cells. [EU]

Esterification: The process of converting an acid into an alkyl or aryl derivative. Most frequently the process consists of the reaction of an acid with an alcohol in the presence of a trace of mineral acid as catalyst or the reaction of an acyl chloride with an alcohol. Esterification can also be accomplished by enzymatic processes. [NIH]

Intestinal: Pertaining to the intestine. [EU]

Iodine: A nonmetallic element of the halogen group that is represented by the atomic symbol I, atomic number 53, and atomic weight of 126.90. It is a nutritionally essential element, especially important in thyroid hormone synthesis. In solution, it has anti-infective properties and is used topically. [NIH]

Neurology: A medical specialty concerned with the study of the structures, functions, and diseases of the nervous system. [NIH]

Niacin: Water-soluble vitamin of the B complex occurring in various animal and plant tissues. Required by the body for the formation of coenzymes NAD and NADP. Has pellagra-curative, vasodilating, and antilipemic properties. [NIH]

Potassium: An element that is in the alkali group of metals. It has an atomic symbol K, atomic number 19, and atomic weight 39.10. It is the chief cation in the intracellular fluid of muscle and other cells. Potassium ion is a strong electrolyte and it plays a significant role in the regulation of fluid volume and maintenance of the water-electrolyte balance. [NIH]

Regeneration: The natural renewal of a structure, as of a lost tissue or part. [EU]

Retinoids: Derivatives of vitamin A. Used clinically in the treatment of severe cystic acne, psoriasis, and other disorders of keratinization. Their possible use in the prophylaxis and treatment of cancer is being actively explored. [NIH]

Rhodopsin: A photoreceptor protein found in retinal rods. It is a complex formed by the binding of retinal, the oxidized form of retinol, to the protein opsin and undergoes a series of complex reactions in response to visible light resulting in the transmission of nerve impulses to the brain. [NIH]

Riboflavin: Nutritional factor found in milk, eggs, malted barley, liver, kidney, heart, and leafy vegetables. The richest natural source is yeast. It occurs in the free form only in the retina of the eye, in whey, and in urine; its principal forms in tissues and cells are as FMN and FAD. [NIH]

Tretinoin: An important regulator of gene expression, particularly during growth and development and in neoplasms. Retinoic acid derived from maternal vitamin A is essential for normal gene expression during embryonic development and either a deficiency or an excess can be teratogenic. It is also a topical dermatologic agent which is used in the treatment of psoriasis, acne vulgaris, and several other skin diseases. It has also been approved for use in promyelocytic leukemia. [NIH]

APPENDIX D. FINDING MEDICAL LIBRARIES

Overview

At a medical library you can find medical texts and reference books, consumer health publications, specialty newspapers and magazines, as well as medical journals. In this Appendix, we show you how to quickly find a medical library in your area.

Preparation

Before going to the library, highlight the references mentioned in this sourcebook that you find interesting. Focus on those items that are not available via the Internet, and ask the reference librarian for help with your search. He or she may know of additional resources that could be helpful to you. Most importantly, your local public library and medical libraries have Interlibrary Loan programs with the National Library of Medicine (NLM), one of the largest medical collections in the world. According to the NLM, most of the literature in the general and historical collections of the National Library of Medicine is available on interlibrary loan to any library. NLM's interlibrary loan services are only available to libraries. If you would like to access NLM medical literature, then visit a library in your area that can request the publications for you.[50]

---

[50] Adapted from the NLM: http://www.nlm.nih.gov/psd/cas/interlibrary.html.

Finding a Local Medical Library

The quickest method to locate medical libraries is to use the Internet-based directory published by the National Network of Libraries of Medicine (NN/LM). This network includes 4626 members and affiliates that provide many services to librarians, health professionals, and the public. To find a library in your area, simply visit **http://nnlm.gov/members/adv.html** or call 1-800-338-7657.

Medical Libraries Open to the Public

In addition to the NN/LM, the National Library of Medicine (NLM) lists a number of libraries that are generally open to the public and have reference facilities. The following is the NLM's list plus hyperlinks to each library Web site. These Web pages can provide information on hours of operation and other restrictions. The list below is a small sample of libraries recommended by the National Library of Medicine (sorted alphabetically by name of the U.S. state or Canadian province where the library is located):[51]

- **Alabama:** Health InfoNet of Jefferson County (Jefferson County Library Cooperative, Lister Hill Library of the Health Sciences), **http://www.uab.edu/infonet/**

- **Alabama:** Richard M. Scrushy Library (American Sports Medicine Institute), **http://www.asmi.org/LIBRARY.HTM**

- **Arizona:** Samaritan Regional Medical Center: The Learning Center (Samaritan Health System, Phoenix, Arizona), **http://www.samaritan.edu/library/bannerlibs.htm**

- **California:** Kris Kelly Health Information Center (St. Joseph Health System), **http://www.humboldt1.com/~kkhic/index.html**

- **California:** Community Health Library of Los Gatos (Community Health Library of Los Gatos), **http://www.healthlib.org/orgresources.html**

- **California:** Consumer Health Program and Services (CHIPS) (County of Los Angeles Public Library, Los Angeles County Harbor-UCLA Medical Center Library) - Carson, CA, **http://www.colapublib.org/services/chips.html**

- **California:** Gateway Health Library (Sutter Gould Medical Foundation)

- **California:** Health Library (Stanford University Medical Center), **http://www-med.stanford.edu/healthlibrary/**

---

[51] Abstracted from **http://www.nlm.nih.gov/medlineplus/libraries.html**

- **California:** Patient Education Resource Center - Health Information and Resources (University of California, San Francisco), **http://sfghdean.ucsf.edu/barnett/PERC/default.asp**

- **California:** Redwood Health Library (Petaluma Health Care District), **http://www.phcd.org/rdwdlib.html**

- **California:** San José PlaneTree Health Library, **http://planetreesanjose.org/**

- **California:** Sutter Resource Library (Sutter Hospitals Foundation), **http://go.sutterhealth.org/comm/resc-library/sac-resources.html**

- **California:** University of California, Davis. Health Sciences Libraries

- **California:** ValleyCare Health Library & Ryan Comer Cancer Resource Center (ValleyCare Health System), **http://www.valleycare.com/library.html**

- **California:** Washington Community Health Resource Library (Washington Community Health Resource Library), **http://www.healthlibrary.org/**

- **Colorado:** William V. Gervasini Memorial Library (Exempla Healthcare), **http://www.exempla.org/conslib.htm**

- **Connecticut:** Hartford Hospital Health Science Libraries (Hartford Hospital), **http://www.harthosp.org/library/**

- **Connecticut:** Healthnet: Connecticut Consumer Health Information Center (University of Connecticut Health Center, Lyman Maynard Stowe Library), **http://library.uchc.edu/departm/hnet/**

- **Connecticut:** Waterbury Hospital Health Center Library (Waterbury Hospital), **http://www.waterburyhospital.com/library/consumer.shtml**

- **Delaware:** Consumer Health Library (Christiana Care Health System, Eugene du Pont Preventive Medicine & Rehabilitation Institute), **http://www.christianacare.org/health_guide/health_guide_pmri_health _info.cfm**

- **Delaware:** Lewis B. Flinn Library (Delaware Academy of Medicine), **http://www.delamed.org/chls.html**

- **Georgia:** Family Resource Library (Medical College of Georgia), **http://cmc.mcg.edu/kids_families/fam_resources/fam_res_lib/frl.htm**

- **Georgia:** Health Resource Center (Medical Center of Central Georgia), **http://www.mccg.org/hrc/hrchome.asp**

- **Hawaii:** Hawaii Medical Library: Consumer Health Information Service (Hawaii Medical Library), **http://hml.org/CHIS/**

- **Idaho:** DeArmond Consumer Health Library (Kootenai Medical Center), http://www.nicon.org/DeArmond/index.htm

- **Illinois:** Health Learning Center of Northwestern Memorial Hospital (Northwestern Memorial Hospital, Health Learning Center), http://www.nmh.org/health_info/hlc.html

- **Illinois:** Medical Library (OSF Saint Francis Medical Center), http://www.osfsaintfrancis.org/general/library/

- **Kentucky:** Medical Library - Services for Patients, Families, Students & the Public (Central Baptist Hospital), http://www.centralbap.com/education/community/library.htm

- **Kentucky:** University of Kentucky - Health Information Library (University of Kentucky, Chandler Medical Center, Health Information Library), http://www.mc.uky.edu/PatientEd/

- **Louisiana:** Alton Ochsner Medical Foundation Library (Alton Ochsner Medical Foundation), http://www.ochsner.org/library/

- **Louisiana:** Louisiana State University Health Sciences Center Medical Library-Shreveport, http://lib-sh.lsuhsc.edu/

- **Maine:** Franklin Memorial Hospital Medical Library (Franklin Memorial Hospital), http://www.fchn.org/fmh/lib.htm

- **Maine:** Gerrish-True Health Sciences Library (Central Maine Medical Center), http://www.cmmc.org/library/library.html

- **Maine:** Hadley Parrot Health Science Library (Eastern Maine Healthcare), http://www.emh.org/hll/hpl/guide.htm

- **Maine:** Maine Medical Center Library (Maine Medical Center), http://www.mmc.org/library/

- **Maine:** Parkview Hospital, http://www.parkviewhospital.org/communit.htm#Library

- **Maine:** Southern Maine Medical Center Health Sciences Library (Southern Maine Medical Center), http://www.smmc.org/services/service.php3?choice=10

- **Maine:** Stephens Memorial Hospital Health Information Library (Western Maine Health), http://www.wmhcc.com/hil_frame.html

- **Manitoba, Canada:** Consumer & Patient Health Information Service (University of Manitoba Libraries), http://www.umanitoba.ca/libraries/units/health/reference/chis.html

- **Manitoba, Canada:** J.W. Crane Memorial Library (Deer Lodge Centre), http://www.deerlodge.mb.ca/library/libraryservices.shtml

- **Maryland:** Health Information Center at the Wheaton Regional Library (Montgomery County, Md., Dept. of Public Libraries, Wheaton Regional Library), **http://www.mont.lib.md.us/healthinfo/hic.asp**

- **Massachusetts:** Baystate Medical Center Library (Baystate Health System), **http://www.baystatehealth.com/1024/**

- **Massachusetts:** Boston University Medical Center Alumni Medical Library (Boston University Medical Center), **http://med-libwww.bu.edu/library/lib.html**

- **Massachusetts:** Lowell General Hospital Health Sciences Library (Lowell General Hospital), **http://www.lowellgeneral.org/library/HomePageLinks/WWW.htm**

- **Massachusetts:** Paul E. Woodard Health Sciences Library (New England Baptist Hospital), **http://www.nebh.org/health_lib.asp**

- **Massachusetts:** St. Luke's Hospital Health Sciences Library (St. Luke's Hospital), **http://www.southcoast.org/library/**

- **Massachusetts:** Treadwell Library Consumer Health Reference Center (Massachusetts General Hospital), **http://www.mgh.harvard.edu/library/chrcindex.html**

- **Massachusetts:** UMass HealthNet (University of Massachusetts Medical School), **http://healthnet.umassmed.edu/**

- **Michigan:** Botsford General Hospital Library - Consumer Health (Botsford General Hospital, Library & Internet Services), **http://www.botsfordlibrary.org/consumer.htm**

- **Michigan:** Helen DeRoy Medical Library (Providence Hospital and Medical Centers), **http://www.providence-hospital.org/library/**

- **Michigan:** Marquette General Hospital - Consumer Health Library (Marquette General Hospital, Health Information Center), **http://www.mgh.org/center.html**

- **Michigan:** Patient Education Resouce Center - University of Michigan Cancer Center (University of Michigan Comprehensive Cancer Center), **http://www.cancer.med.umich.edu/learn/leares.htm**

- **Michigan:** Sladen Library & Center for Health Information Resources - Consumer Health Information, **http://www.sladen.hfhs.org/library/consumer/index.html**

- **Montana:** Center for Health Information (St. Patrick Hospital and Health Sciences Center), **http://www.saintpatrick.org/chi/librarydetail.php3?ID=41**

- **National:** Consumer Health Library Directory (Medical Library Association, Consumer and Patient Health Information Section), http://caphis.mlanet.org/directory/index.html

- **National:** National Network of Libraries of Medicine (National Library of Medicine) - provides library services for health professionals in the United States who do not have access to a medical library, http://nnlm.gov/

- **National:** NN/LM List of Libraries Serving the Public (National Network of Libraries of Medicine), http://nnlm.gov/members/

- **Nevada:** Health Science Library, West Charleston Library (Las Vegas Clark County Library District), http://www.lvccld.org/special_collections/medical/index.htm

- **New Hampshire:** Dartmouth Biomedical Libraries (Dartmouth College Library), http://www.dartmouth.edu/~biomed/resources.htmld/conshealth.htmld/

- **New Jersey:** Consumer Health Library (Rahway Hospital), http://www.rahwayhospital.com/library.htm

- **New Jersey:** Dr. Walter Phillips Health Sciences Library (Englewood Hospital and Medical Center), http://www.englewoodhospital.com/links/index.htm

- **New Jersey:** Meland Foundation (Englewood Hospital and Medical Center), http://www.geocities.com/ResearchTriangle/9360/

- **New York:** Choices in Health Information (New York Public Library) - NLM Consumer Pilot Project participant, http://www.nypl.org/branch/health/links.html

- **New York:** Health Information Center (Upstate Medical University, State University of New York), http://www.upstate.edu/library/hic/

- **New York:** Health Sciences Library (Long Island Jewish Medical Center), http://www.lij.edu/library/library.html

- **New York:** ViaHealth Medical Library (Rochester General Hospital), http://www.nyam.org/library/

- **Ohio:** Consumer Health Library (Akron General Medical Center, Medical & Consumer Health Library), http://www.akrongeneral.org/hwlibrary.htm

- **Oklahoma:** Saint Francis Health System Patient/Family Resource Center (Saint Francis Health System), http://www.sfh-tulsa.com/patientfamilycenter/default.asp

- **Oregon:** Planetree Health Resource Center (Mid-Columbia Medical Center), **http://www.mcmc.net/phrc/**

- **Pennsylvania:** Community Health Information Library (Milton S. Hershey Medical Center), **http://www.hmc.psu.edu/commhealth/**

- **Pennsylvania:** Community Health Resource Library (Geisinger Medical Center), **http://www.geisinger.edu/education/commlib.shtml**

- **Pennsylvania:** HealthInfo Library (Moses Taylor Hospital), **http://www.mth.org/healthwellness.html**

- **Pennsylvania:** Hopwood Library (University of Pittsburgh, Health Sciences Library System), **http://www.hsls.pitt.edu/chi/hhrcinfo.html**

- **Pennsylvania:** Koop Community Health Information Center (College of Physicians of Philadelphia), **http://www.collphyphil.org/kooppg1.shtml**

- **Pennsylvania:** Learning Resources Center - Medical Library (Susquehanna Health System), **http://www.shscares.org/services/lrc/index.asp**

- **Pennsylvania:** Medical Library (UPMC Health System), **http://www.upmc.edu/passavant/library.htm**

- **Quebec, Canada:** Medical Library (Montreal General Hospital), **http://ww2.mcgill.ca/mghlib/**

- **South Dakota:** Rapid City Regional Hospital - Health Information Center (Rapid City Regional Hospital, Health Information Center), **http://www.rcrh.org/education/LibraryResourcesConsumers.htm**

- **Texas:** Houston HealthWays (Houston Academy of Medicine-Texas Medical Center Library), **http://hhw.library.tmc.edu/**

- **Texas:** Matustik Family Resource Center (Cook Children's Health Care System), **http://www.cookchildrens.com/Matustik_Library.html**

- **Washington:** Community Health Library (Kittitas Valley Community Hospital), **http://www.kvch.com/**

- **Washington:** Southwest Washington Medical Center Library (Southwest Washington Medical Center), **http://www.swmedctr.com/Home/**

APPENDIX E. YOUR RIGHTS AND INSURANCE

Overview

Any patient with vitiligo faces a series of issues related more to the healthcare industry than to the medical condition itself. This appendix covers two important topics in this regard: your rights and responsibilities as a patient, and how to get the most out of your medical insurance plan.

Your Rights as a Patient

The President's Advisory Commission on Consumer Protection and Quality in the Healthcare Industry has created the following summary of your rights as a patient.[52]

Information Disclosure

Consumers have the right to receive accurate, easily understood information. Some consumers require assistance in making informed decisions about health plans, health professionals, and healthcare facilities. Such information includes:

- *Health plans.* Covered benefits, cost-sharing, and procedures for resolving complaints, licensure, certification, and accreditation status, comparable measures of quality and consumer satisfaction, provider network composition, the procedures that govern access to specialists and emergency services, and care management information.

---

[52]Adapted from Consumer Bill of Rights and Responsibilities: **http://www.hcqualitycommission.gov/press/cbor.html#head1**.

- *Health professionals.* Education, board certification, and recertification, years of practice, experience performing certain procedures, and comparable measures of quality and consumer satisfaction.

- *Healthcare facilities.* Experience in performing certain procedures and services, accreditation status, comparable measures of quality, worker, and consumer satisfaction, and procedures for resolving complaints.

- *Consumer assistance programs.* Programs must be carefully structured to promote consumer confidence and to work cooperatively with health plans, providers, payers, and regulators. Desirable characteristics of such programs are sponsorship that ensures accountability to the interests of consumers and stable, adequate funding.

Choice of Providers and Plans

Consumers have the right to a choice of healthcare providers that is sufficient to ensure access to appropriate high-quality healthcare. To ensure such choice, the Commission recommends the following:

- *Provider network adequacy.* All health plan networks should provide access to sufficient numbers and types of providers to assure that all covered services will be accessible without unreasonable delay -- including access to emergency services 24 hours a day and 7 days a week. If a health plan has an insufficient number or type of providers to provide a covered benefit with the appropriate degree of specialization, the plan should ensure that the consumer obtains the benefit outside the network at no greater cost than if the benefit were obtained from participating providers.

- *Women's health services.* Women should be able to choose a qualified provider offered by a plan -- such as gynecologists, certified nurse midwives, and other qualified healthcare providers -- for the provision of covered care necessary to provide routine and preventative women's healthcare services.

- *Access to specialists.* Consumers with complex or serious medical conditions who require frequent specialty care should have direct access to a qualified specialist of their choice within a plan's network of providers. Authorizations, when required, should be for an adequate number of direct access visits under an approved treatment plan.

- *Transitional care.* Consumers who are undergoing a course of treatment for a chronic or disabling condition (or who are in the second or third trimester of a pregnancy) at the time they involuntarily change health plans or at a time when a provider is terminated by a plan for other than cause should be able to continue seeing their current specialty providers for up to 90 days (or through completion of postpartum care) to allow for transition of care.

- *Choice of health plans.* Public and private group purchasers should, wherever feasible, offer consumers a choice of high-quality health insurance plans.

Access to Emergency Services

Consumers have the right to access emergency healthcare services when and where the need arises. Health plans should provide payment when a consumer presents to an emergency department with acute symptoms of sufficient severity--including severe pain--such that a "prudent layperson" could reasonably expect the absence of medical attention to result in placing that consumer's health in serious jeopardy, serious impairment to bodily functions, or serious dysfunction of any bodily organ or part.

Participation in Treatment Decisions

Consumers have the right and responsibility to fully participate in all decisions related to their healthcare. Consumers who are unable to fully participate in treatment decisions have the right to be represented by parents, guardians, family members, or other conservators. Physicians and other health professionals should:

- Provide patients with sufficient information and opportunity to decide among treatment options consistent with the informed consent process.

- Discuss all treatment options with a patient in a culturally competent manner, including the option of no treatment at all.

- Ensure that persons with disabilities have effective communications with members of the health system in making such decisions.

- Discuss all current treatments a consumer may be undergoing.

- Discuss all risks, benefits, and consequences to treatment or nontreatment.

- Give patients the opportunity to refuse treatment and to express preferences about future treatment decisions.

- Discuss the use of advance directives -- both living wills and durable powers of attorney for healthcare -- with patients and their designated family members.

- Abide by the decisions made by their patients and/or their designated representatives consistent with the informed consent process.

Health plans, health providers, and healthcare facilities should:

- Disclose to consumers factors -- such as methods of compensation, ownership of or interest in healthcare facilities, or matters of conscience -- that could influence advice or treatment decisions.

- Assure that provider contracts do not contain any so-called "gag clauses" or other contractual mechanisms that restrict healthcare providers' ability to communicate with and advise patients about medically necessary treatment options.

- Be prohibited from penalizing or seeking retribution against healthcare professionals or other health workers for advocating on behalf of their patients.

Respect and Nondiscrimination

Consumers have the right to considerate, respectful care from all members of the healthcare industry at all times and under all circumstances. An environment of mutual respect is essential to maintain a quality healthcare system. To assure that right, the Commission recommends the following:

- Consumers must not be discriminated against in the delivery of healthcare services consistent with the benefits covered in their policy, or as required by law, based on race, ethnicity, national origin, religion, sex, age, mental or physical disability, sexual orientation, genetic information, or source of payment.

- Consumers eligible for coverage under the terms and conditions of a health plan or program, or as required by law, must not be discriminated against in marketing and enrollment practices based on race, ethnicity, national origin, religion, sex, age, mental or physical disability, sexual orientation, genetic information, or source of payment.

Confidentiality of Health Information

Consumers have the right to communicate with healthcare providers in confidence and to have the confidentiality of their individually identifiable healthcare information protected. Consumers also have the right to review and copy their own medical records and request amendments to their records.

Complaints and Appeals

Consumers have the right to a fair and efficient process for resolving differences with their health plans, healthcare providers, and the institutions that serve them, including a rigorous system of internal review and an independent system of external review. A free copy of the Patient's Bill of Rights is available from the American Hospital Association.[53]

Patient Responsibilities

Treatment is a two-way street between you and your healthcare providers. To underscore the importance of finance in modern healthcare as well as your responsibility for the financial aspects of your care, the President's Advisory Commission on Consumer Protection and Quality in the Healthcare Industry has proposed that patients understand the following "Consumer Responsibilities."[54] In a healthcare system that protects consumers' rights, it is reasonable to expect and encourage consumers to assume certain responsibilities. Greater individual involvement by the consumer in his or her care increases the likelihood of achieving the best outcome and helps support a quality-oriented, cost-conscious environment. Such responsibilities include:

- Take responsibility for maximizing healthy habits such as exercising, not smoking, and eating a healthy diet.

- Work collaboratively with healthcare providers in developing and carrying out agreed-upon treatment plans.

- Disclose relevant information and clearly communicate wants and needs.

- Use your health insurance plan's internal complaint and appeal processes to address your concerns.

- Avoid knowingly spreading disease.

---

[53] To order your free copy of the Patient's Bill of Rights, telephone 312-422-3000 or visit the American Hospital Association's Web site: http://www.aha.org. Click on "Resource Center," go to "Search" at bottom of page, and then type in "Patient's Bill of Rights." The Patient's Bill of Rights is also available from Fax on Demand, at 312-422-2020, document number 471124.

[54] Adapted from http://www.hcqualitycommission.gov/press/cbor.html#head1.

- Recognize the reality of risks, the limits of the medical science, and the human fallibility of the healthcare professional.

- Be aware of a healthcare provider's obligation to be reasonably efficient and equitable in providing care to other patients and the community.

- Become knowledgeable about your health plan's coverage and options (when available) including all covered benefits, limitations, and exclusions, rules regarding use of network providers, coverage and referral rules, appropriate processes to secure additional information, and the process to appeal coverage decisions.

- Show respect for other patients and health workers.

- Make a good-faith effort to meet financial obligations.

- Abide by administrative and operational procedures of health plans, healthcare providers, and Government health benefit programs.

Choosing an Insurance Plan

There are a number of official government agencies that help consumers understand their healthcare insurance choices.[55] The U.S. Department of Labor, in particular, recommends ten ways to make your health benefits choices work best for you.[56]

1. Your options are important. There are many different types of health benefit plans. Find out which one your employer offers, then check out the plan, or plans, offered. Your employer's human resource office, the health plan administrator, or your union can provide information to help you match your needs and preferences with the available plans. The more information you have, the better your healthcare decisions will be.

2. Reviewing the benefits available. Do the plans offered cover preventive care, well-baby care, vision or dental care? Are there deductibles? Answers to these questions can help determine the out-of-pocket expenses you may face. Matching your needs and those of your family members will result in the best possible benefits. Cheapest may not always be best. Your goal is high quality health benefits.

---

[55] More information about quality across programs is provided at the following AHRQ Web site:
http://www.ahrq.gov/consumer/qntascii/qnthplan.htm .
[56] Adapted from the Department of Labor:
http://www.dol.gov/dol/pwba/public/pubs/health/top10-text.html.

3. Look for quality. The quality of healthcare services varies, but quality can be measured. You should consider the quality of healthcare in deciding among the healthcare plans or options available to you. Not all health plans, doctors, hospitals and other providers give the highest quality care. Fortunately, there is quality information you can use right now to help you compare your healthcare choices. Find out how you can measure quality. Consult the U.S. Department of Health and Human Services publication "Your Guide to Choosing Quality Health Care" on the Internet at **www.ahcpr.gov/consumer**.

4. Your plan's summary plan description (SPD) provides a wealth of information. Your health plan administrator can provide you with a copy of your plan's SPD. It outlines your benefits and your legal rights under the Employee Retirement Income Security Act (ERISA), the federal law that protects your health benefits. It should contain information about the coverage of dependents, what services will require a co-pay, and the circumstances under which your employer can change or terminate a health benefits plan. Save the SPD and all other health plan brochures and documents, along with memos or correspondence from your employer relating to health benefits.

5. Assess your benefit coverage as your family status changes. Marriage, divorce, childbirth or adoption, and the death of a spouse are all life events that may signal a need to change your health benefits. You, your spouse and dependent children may be eligible for a special enrollment period under provisions of the Health Insurance Portability and Accountability Act (HIPAA). Even without life-changing events, the information provided by your employer should tell you how you can change benefits or switch plans, if more than one plan is offered. If your spouse's employer also offers a health benefits package, consider coordinating both plans for maximum coverage.

6. Changing jobs and other life events can affect your health benefits. Under the Consolidated Omnibus Budget Reconciliation Act (COBRA), you, your covered spouse, and your dependent children may be eligible to purchase extended health coverage under your employer's plan if you lose your job, change employers, get divorced, or upon occurrence of certain other events. Coverage can range from 18 to 36 months depending on your situation. COBRA applies to most employers with 20 or more workers and requires your plan to notify you of your rights. Most plans require eligible individuals to make their COBRA election within 60 days of the plan's notice. Be sure to follow up with your plan sponsor if you don't receive notice, and make sure you respond within the allotted time.

7. HIPAA can also help if you are changing jobs, particularly if you have a medical condition. HIPAA generally limits pre-existing condition exclusions to a maximum of 12 months (18 months for late enrollees). HIPAA also requires this maximum period to be reduced by the length of time you had prior "creditable coverage." You should receive a certificate documenting your prior creditable coverage from your old plan when coverage ends.

8. Plan for retirement. Before you retire, find out what health benefits, if any, extend to you and your spouse during your retirement years. Consult with your employer's human resources office, your union, the plan administrator, and check your SPD. Make sure there is no conflicting information among these sources about the benefits you will receive or the circumstances under which they can change or be eliminated. With this information in hand, you can make other important choices, like finding out if you are eligible for Medicare and Medigap insurance coverage.

9. Know how to file an appeal if your health benefits claim is denied. Understand how your plan handles grievances and where to make appeals of the plan's decisions. Keep records and copies of correspondence. Check your health benefits package and your SPD to determine who is responsible for handling problems with benefit claims. Contact PWBA for customer service assistance if you are unable to obtain a response to your complaint.

10. You can take steps to improve the quality of the healthcare and the health benefits you receive. Look for and use things like Quality Reports and Accreditation Reports whenever you can. Quality reports may contain consumer ratings -- how satisfied consumers are with the doctors in their plan, for instance-- and clinical performance measures -- how well a healthcare organization prevents and treats illness. Accreditation reports provide information on how accredited organizations meet national standards, and often include clinical performance measures. Look for these quality measures whenever possible. Consult "Your Guide to Choosing Quality Health Care" on the Internet at **www.ahcpr.gov/consumer**.

Medicare and Medicaid

Illness strikes both rich and poor families. For low-income families, Medicaid is available to defer the costs of treatment. The Health Care Financing Administration (HCFA) administers Medicare, the nation's largest health insurance program, which covers 39 million Americans. In the following pages, you will learn the basics about Medicare insurance as well as useful contact information on how to find more in-depth information about Medicaid.[57]

Who is Eligible for Medicare?

Generally, you are eligible for Medicare if you or your spouse worked for at least 10 years in Medicare-covered employment and you are 65 years old and a citizen or permanent resident of the United States. You might also qualify for coverage if you are under age 65 but have a disability or End-Stage Renal disease (permanent kidney failure requiring dialysis or transplant). Here are some simple guidelines:

You can get Part A at age 65 without having to pay premiums if:

- You are already receiving retirement benefits from Social Security or the Railroad Retirement Board.

- You are eligible to receive Social Security or Railroad benefits but have not yet filed for them.

- You or your spouse had Medicare-covered government employment.

If you are under 65, you can get Part A without having to pay premiums if:

- You have received Social Security or Railroad Retirement Board disability benefit for 24 months.

- You are a kidney dialysis or kidney transplant patient.

Medicare has two parts:

- Part A (Hospital Insurance). Most people do not have to pay for Part A.
- Part B (Medical Insurance). Most people pay monthly for Part B.

Part A (Hospital Insurance)

Helps Pay For: Inpatient hospital care, care in critical access hospitals (small facilities that give limited outpatient and inpatient services to people in rural areas) and skilled nursing facilities, hospice care, and some home healthcare.

---

[57] This section has been adapted from the Official U.S. Site for Medicare Information: **http://www.medicare.gov/Basics/Overview.asp**.

Cost: Most people get Part A automatically when they turn age 65. You do not have to pay a monthly payment called a premium for Part A because you or a spouse paid Medicare taxes while you were working.

If you (or your spouse) did not pay Medicare taxes while you were working and you are age 65 or older, you still may be able to buy Part A. If you are not sure you have Part A, look on your red, white, and blue Medicare card. It will show "Hospital Part A" on the lower left corner of the card. You can also call the Social Security Administration toll free at 1-800-772-1213 or call your local Social Security office for more information about buying Part A. If you get benefits from the Railroad Retirement Board, call your local RRB office or 1-800-808-0772. For more information, call your Fiscal Intermediary about Part A bills and services. The phone number for the Fiscal Intermediary office in your area can be obtained from the following Web site: **http://www.medicare.gov/Contacts/home.asp**.

Part B (Medical Insurance)

Helps Pay For: Doctors, services, outpatient hospital care, and some other medical services that Part A does not cover, such as the services of physical and occupational therapists, and some home healthcare. Part B helps pay for covered services and supplies when they are medically necessary.

Cost: As of 2001, you pay the Medicare Part B premium of $50.00 per month. In some cases this amount may be higher if you did not choose Part B when you first became eligible at age 65. The cost of Part B may go up 10% for each 12-month period that you were eligible for Part B but declined coverage, except in special cases. You will have to pay the extra 10% cost for the rest of your life.

Enrolling in Part B is your choice. You can sign up for Part B anytime during a 7-month period that begins 3 months before you turn 65. Visit your local Social Security office, or call the Social Security Administration at 1-800-772-1213 to sign up. If you choose to enroll in Part B, the premium is usually taken out of your monthly Social Security, Railroad Retirement, or Civil Service Retirement payment. If you do not receive any of the above payments, Medicare sends you a bill for your part B premium every 3 months. You should receive your Medicare premium bill in the mail by the 10th of the month. If you do not, call the Social Security Administration at 1-800-772-1213, or your local Social Security office. If you get benefits from the Railroad Retirement Board, call your local RRB office or 1-800-808-0772. For more information, call your Medicare carrier about bills and services. The phone number for the Medicare carrier in your area can be found at the following Web site: **http://www.medicare.gov/Contacts/home.asp**. You may have choices in how you get your healthcare including the Original Medicare Plan, Medicare Managed Care Plans (like HMOs), and Medicare Private Fee-for-Service Plans.

Medicaid

Medicaid is a joint federal and state program that helps pay medical costs for some people with low incomes and limited resources. Medicaid programs vary from state to state. People on Medicaid may also get coverage for nursing home care and outpatient prescription drugs which are not covered by Medicare. You can find more information about Medicaid on the HCFA.gov Web site at **http://www.hcfa.gov/medicaid/medicaid.htm**.

States also have programs that pay some or all of Medicare's premiums and may also pay Medicare deductibles and coinsurance for certain people who have Medicare and a low income. To qualify, you must have:

- Part A (Hospital Insurance),

- Assets, such as bank accounts, stocks, and bonds that are not more than $4,000 for a single person, or $6,000 for a couple, and

- A monthly income that is below certain limits.

For more information on these programs, look at the Medicare Savings Programs brochure, **http://www.medicare.gov/Library/PDFNavigation/PDFInterim.asp?Language=English&Type=Pub&PubID=10126**. There are also Prescription Drug Assistance Programs available. Find information on these programs which offer discounts or free medications to individuals in need at **http://www.medicare.gov/Prescription/Home.asp**.

NORD's Medication Assistance Programs

Finally, the National Organization for Rare Disorders, Inc. (NORD) administers medication programs sponsored by humanitarian-minded pharmaceutical and biotechnology companies to help uninsured or under-insured individuals secure life-saving or life-sustaining drugs.[58] NORD

---

[58] Adapted from NORD: **http://www.rarediseases.org/cgi-bin/nord/progserv#patient?id=rPIzL9oD&mv_pc=30**.

programs ensure that certain vital drugs are available "to those individuals whose income is too high to qualify for Medicaid but too low to pay for their prescribed medications." The program has standards for fairness, equity, and unbiased eligibility. It currently covers some 14 programs for nine pharmaceutical companies. NORD also offers early access programs for investigational new drugs (IND) under the approved "Treatment INDs" programs of the Food and Drug Administration (FDA). In these programs, a limited number of individuals can receive investigational drugs that have yet to be approved by the FDA. These programs are generally designed for rare diseases or disorders. For more information, visit **www.rarediseases.org**.

Additional Resources

In addition to the references already listed in this chapter, you may need more information on health insurance, hospitals, or the healthcare system in general. The NIH has set up an excellent guidance Web site that addresses these and other issues. Topics include:[59]

- Health Insurance:
  http://www.nlm.nih.gov/medlineplus/healthinsurance.html

- Health Statistics:
  http://www.nlm.nih.gov/medlineplus/healthstatistics.html

- HMO and Managed Care:
  http://www.nlm.nih.gov/medlineplus/managedcare.html

- Hospice Care: **http://www.nlm.nih.gov/medlineplus/hospicecare.html**

- Medicaid: **http://www.nlm.nih.gov/medlineplus/medicaid.html**

- Medicare: **http://www.nlm.nih.gov/medlineplus/medicare.html**

- Nursing Homes and Long-term Care:
  http://www.nlm.nih.gov/medlineplus/nursinghomes.html

- Patient's Rights, Confidentiality, Informed Consent, Ombudsman Programs, Privacy and Patient Issues:
  http://www.nlm.nih.gov/medlineplus/patientissues.html

---

[59] You can access this information at:
http://www.nlm.nih.gov/medlineplus/healthsystem.html.

ONLINE GLOSSARIES

The Internet provides access to a number of free-to-use medical dictionaries and glossaries. The National Library of Medicine has compiled the following list of online dictionaries:

- ADAM Medical Encyclopedia (A.D.A.M., Inc.), comprehensive medical reference: **http://www.nlm.nih.gov/medlineplus/encyclopedia.html**

- MedicineNet.com Medical Dictionary (MedicineNet, Inc.): **http://www.medterms.com/Script/Main/hp.asp**

- Merriam-Webster Medical Dictionary (Inteli-Health, Inc.): **http://www.intelihealth.com/IH/**

- Multilingual Glossary of Technical and Popular Medical Terms in Eight European Languages (European Commission) - Danish, Dutch, English, French, German, Italian, Portuguese, and Spanish: **http://allserv.rug.ac.be/~rvdstich/eugloss/welcome.html**

- On-line Medical Dictionary (CancerWEB): **http://www.graylab.ac.uk/omd/**

- Technology Glossary (National Library of Medicine) - Health Care Technology: **http://www.nlm.nih.gov/nichsr/ta101/ta10108.htm**

- Terms and Definitions (Office of Rare Diseases): **http://rarediseases.info.nih.gov/ord/glossary_a-e.html**

Beyond these, MEDLINEplus contains a very user-friendly encyclopedia covering every aspect of medicine (licensed from A.D.A.M., Inc.). The ADAM Medical Encyclopedia Web site address is **http://www.nlm.nih.gov/medlineplus/encyclopedia.html**. ADAM is also available on commercial Web sites such as Web MD (**http://my.webmd.com/adam/asset/adam_disease_articles/a_to_z/a**) and drkoop.com (**http://www.drkoop.com/**). Topics of interest can be researched by using keywords before continuing elsewhere, as these basic definitions and concepts will be useful in more advanced areas of research. You may choose to print various pages specifically relating to vitiligo and keep them on file. The NIH, in particular, suggests that patients with vitiligo visit the following Web sites in the ADAM Medical Encyclopedia:

- **Basic Guidelines for Diseasex**

  Vitiligo
  Web site:
  http://www.nlm.nih.gov/medlineplus/ency/article/000831.htm

- **Signs & Symptoms for Diseasex**

  Hyperpigmentation
  Web site:
  http://www.nlm.nih.gov/medlineplus/ency/article/003242.htm

  Sunburn
  Web site:
  http://www.nlm.nih.gov/medlineplus/ency/article/003227.htm

  Telangiectasia
  Web site:
  http://www.nlm.nih.gov/medlineplus/ency/article/003284.htm

- **Diagnostics and Tests for Diseasex**

  Biopsy
  Web site:
  http://www.nlm.nih.gov/medlineplus/ency/article/003416.htm

  CBC
  Web site:
  http://www.nlm.nih.gov/medlineplus/ency/article/003642.htm

  Skin biopsy
  Web site:
  http://www.nlm.nih.gov/medlineplus/ency/article/003840.htm

  TSH
  Web site:
  http://www.nlm.nih.gov/medlineplus/ency/article/003684.htm

- **Background Topics for Diseasex**

Incidence
Web site:
http://www.nlm.nih.gov/medlineplus/ency/article/002387.htm

Systemic
Web site:
http://www.nlm.nih.gov/medlineplus/ency/article/002294.htm

Online Dictionary Directories

The following are additional online directories compiled by the National Library of Medicine, including a number of specialized medical dictionaries and glossaries:

- Medical Dictionaries: Medical & Biological (World Health Organization): **http://www.who.int/hlt/virtuallibrary/English/diction.htm#Medical**

- MEL-Michigan Electronic Library List of Online Health and Medical Dictionaries (Michigan Electronic Library): **http://mel.lib.mi.us/health/health-dictionaries.html**

- Patient Education: Glossaries (DMOZ Open Directory Project): **http://dmoz.org/Health/Education/Patient_Education/Glossaries/**

- Web of Online Dictionaries (Bucknell University): **http://www.yourdictionary.com/diction5.html#medicine**

VITILIGO GLOSSARY

The following is a complete glossary of terms used in this sourcebook. The definitions are derived from official public sources including the National Institutes of Health [NIH] and the European Union [EU]. After this glossary, we list a number of additional hardbound and electronic glossaries and dictionaries that you may wish to consult.

Aberrant: Wandering or deviating from the usual or normal course. [EU]

Acrodermatitis: Inflammation involving the skin of the extremities, especially the hands and feet. Several forms are known, some idiopathic and some hereditary. The infantile form is called Gianotti-Crosti syndrome. [NIH]

ACTH: Adrenocorticotropic hormone. [EU]

Albinism: General term for a number of inherited defects of amino acid metabolism in which there is a deficiency or absence of pigment in the eyes, skin, or hair. [NIH]

Alkaloid: One of a large group of nitrogenous basis substances found in plants. They are usually very bitter and many are pharmacologically active. Examples are atropine, caffeine, coniine, morphine, nicotine, quinine, strychnine. The term is also applied to synthetic substances (artificial a's) which have structures similar to plant alkaloids, such as procaine. [EU]

Alleles: Mutually exclusive forms of the same gene, occupying the same locus on homologous chromosomes, and governing the same biochemical and developmental process. [NIH]

Allylamine: Possesses an unusual and selective cytotoxicity for vascular smooth muscle cells in dogs and rats. Useful for experiments dealing with arterial injury, myocardial fibrosis or cardiac decompensation. [NIH]

Alopecia: Baldness; absence of the hair from skin areas where it normally is present. [EU]

Analgesic: An agent that alleviates pain without causing loss of consciousness. [EU]

Analogous: Resembling or similar in some respects, as in function or appearance, but not in origin or development;. [EU]

Anemia: A reduction in the number of circulating erythrocytes or in the quantity of hemoglobin. [NIH]

Anesthesia: A state characterized by loss of feeling or sensation. This depression of nerve function is usually the result of pharmacologic action and is induced to allow performance of surgery or other painful procedures. [NIH]

Aniridia: A congenital abnormality in which there is only a rudimentary iris. This is due to the failure of the optic cup to grow. Aniridia also occurs in a hereditary form, usually autosomal dominant. [NIH]

Antigen: Any substance which is capable, under appropriate conditions, of inducing a specific immune response and of reacting with the products of that response, that is, with specific antibody or specifically sensitized T-lymphocytes, or both. Antigens may be soluble substances, such as toxins and foreign proteins, or particulate, such as bacteria and tissue cells; however, only the portion of the protein or polysaccharide molecule known as the antigenic determinant (q.v.) combines with antibody or a specific receptor on a lymphocyte. Abbreviated Ag. [EU]

Antioxidant: One of many widely used synthetic or natural substances added to a product to prevent or delay its deterioration by action of oxygen in the air. Rubber, paints, vegetable oils, and prepared foods commonly contain antioxidants. [EU]

Arginine: An essential amino acid that is physiologically active in the L-form. [NIH]

Assay: Determination of the amount of a particular constituent of a mixture, or of the biological or pharmacological potency of a drug. [EU]

Atopic: Pertaining to an atopen or to atopy; allergic. [EU]

Auditory: Pertaining to the sense of hearing. [EU]

Autoimmunity: Process whereby the immune system reacts against the body's own tissues. Autoimmunity may produce or be caused by autoimmune diseases. [NIH]

Bacteria: Unicellular prokaryotic microorganisms which generally possess rigid cell walls, multiply by cell division, and exhibit three principal forms: round or coccal, rodlike or bacillary, and spiral or spirochetal. [NIH]

Benign: Not malignant; not recurrent; favourable for recovery. [EU]

Biochemical: Relating to biochemistry; characterized by, produced by, or involving chemical reactions in living organisms. [EU]

Biopsy: The removal and examination, usually microscopic, of tissue from the living body, performed to establish precise diagnosis. [EU]

Blindness: The inability to see or the loss or absence of perception of visual stimuli. This condition may be the result of eye diseases; optic nerve diseases; optic chiasm diseases; or brain diseases affecting the visual pathways or occipital lobe. [NIH]

Blister: Visible accumulations of fluid within or beneath the epidermis. [NIH]

Bullous: Pertaining to or characterized by bullae. [EU]

Candidiasis: Infection with a fungus of the genus Candida. It is usually a superficial infection of the moist cutaneous areas of the body, and is generally caused by C. albicans; it most commonly involves the skin (dermatocandidiasis), oral mucous membranes (thrush, def. 1), respiratory tract (bronchocandidiasis), and vagina (vaginitis). Rarely there is a systemic infection or endocarditis. Called also moniliasis, candidosis, oidiomycosis, and formerly blastodendriosis. [EU]

Capsules: Hard or soft soluble containers used for the oral administration of medicine. [NIH]

Carbohydrate: An aldehyde or ketone derivative of a polyhydric alcohol, particularly of the pentahydric and hexahydric alcohols. They are so named because the hydrogen and oxygen are usually in the proportion to form water, $(CH_2O)n$. The most important carbohydrates are the starches, sugars, celluloses, and gums. They are classified into mono-, di-, tri-, poly- and heterosaccharides. [EU]

Carbuncle: An infection of cutaneous and subcutaneous tissue that consists of a cluster of boils. Commonly, the causative agent is staphylococcus AUREUS. Carbuncles produce fever, leukocytosis, extreme pain, and prostration. [NIH]

Carcinoma: A malignant new growth made up of epithelial cells tending to infiltrate the surrounding tissues and give rise to metastases. [EU]

Catalase: An oxidoreductase that catalyzes the conversion of hydrogen peroxide to water and oxygen. It is present in many animal cells. A deficiency of this enzyme results in ACATALASIA. EC 1.11.1.6. [NIH]

Cataract: An opacity, partial or complete, of one or both eyes, on or in the lens or capsule, especially an opacity impairing vision or causing blindness. The many kinds of cataract are classified by their morphology (size, shape, location) or etiology (cause and time of occurrence). [EU]

Catechols: A group of 1,2-benzenediols that contain the general formula R-$C_6H_5O_2$. [NIH]

Cellulitis: An acute, diffuse, and suppurative inflammation of loose connective tissue, particularly the deep subcutaneous tissues, and sometimes muscle, which is most commonly seen as a result of infection of a wound, ulcer, or other skin lesions. [NIH]

Chloroquine: The prototypical antimalarial agent with a mechanism that is not well understood. It has also been used to treat rheumatoid arthritis, systemic lupus erythematosus, and in the systemic therapy of amebic liver abscesses. [NIH]

Cholesterol: The principal sterol of all higher animals, distributed in body tissues, especially the brain and spinal cord, and in animal fats and oils. [NIH]

Choroideremia: An X chromosome-linked abnormality characterized by atrophy of the choroid and degeneration of the retinal pigment epithelium causing night blindness. [NIH]

Chronic: Persisting over a long period of time. [EU]

Clobetasol: Topical corticosteroid that is absorbed faster than fluocinonide. It is used in psoriasis, but may cause marked adrenocortical suppression. [NIH]

Clotrimazole: An imidazole derivative with a broad spectrum of antimycotic activity. It inhibits biosynthesis of the sterol ergostol, an important component of fungal cell membranes. Its action leads to increased membrane permeability and apparent disruption of enzyme systems bound to the membrane. [NIH]

Codeine: An opioid analgesic related to morphine but with less potent analgesic properties and mild sedative effects. It also acts centrally to suppress cough. [NIH]

Colitis: Inflammation of the colon. [EU]

Contracture: A condition of fixed high resistance to passive stretch of a muscle, resulting from fibrosis of the tissues supporting the muscles or the joints, or from disorders of the muscle fibres. [EU]

Cutaneous: Pertaining to the skin; dermal; dermic. [EU]

Cyst: Any closed cavity or sac; normal or abnormal, lined by epithelium, and especially one that contains a liquid or semisolid material. [EU]

Cytokines: Non-antibody proteins secreted by inflammatory leukocytes and some non-leukocytic cells, that act as intercellular mediators. They differ from classical hormones in that they are produced by a number of tissue or cell types rather than by specialized glands. They generally act locally in a paracrine or autocrine rather than endocrine manner. [NIH]

Cytomegalovirus: A genus of the family herpesviridae, subfamily betaherpesvirinae, infecting the salivary glands, liver, spleen, lungs, eyes, and other organs, in which they produce characteristically enlarged cells with intranuclear inclusions. Infection with Cytomegalovirus is also seen as an opportunistic infection in AIDS. [NIH]

Depigmentation: Removal or loss of pigment, especially melanin. [EU]

Dermatology: A medical specialty concerned with the skin, its structure, functions, diseases, and treatment. [NIH]

Dermatophytosis. Any superficial fungal infection caused by a dermatophyte and involving the stratum corneum of the skin, hair, and nails. The term broadly comprises onychophytosis and the various form of tinea (ringworm), sometimes being used specifically to designate tinea pedis (athlete's foot). Called also epidermomycosis. [EU]

Dermatosis: Any skin disease, especially one not characterized by inflammation. [EU]

Diarrhea: Passage of excessively liquid or excessively frequent stools. [NIH]

Didanosine: A dideoxynucleoside compound in which the 3'-hydroxy group on the sugar moiety has been replaced by a hydrogen. This modification prevents the formation of phosphodiester linkages which are needed for the completion of nucleic acid chains. Didanosine is a potent inhibitor of HIV replication, acting as a chain-terminator of viral DNA by binding to reverse transcriptase; ddI is then metabolized to dideoxyadenosine triphosphate, its putative active metabolite. [NIH]

Dyes: Chemical substances that are used to stain and color other materials. The coloring may or may not be permanent. Dyes can also be used as therapeutic agents and test reagents in medicine and scientific research. [NIH]

Dysplasia: Abnormality of development; in pathology, alteration in size, shape, and organization of adult cells. [EU]

Dystonia: Disordered tonicity of muscle. [EU]

Dystrophy: Any disorder arising from defective or faulty nutrition, especially the muscular dystrophies. [EU]

Econazole: A broad spectrum antimycotic with some action against Gram positive bacteria. It is used topically in dermatomycoses also orally and parenterally. [NIH]

Eczema: A pruritic papulovesicular dermatitis occurring as a reaction to many endogenous and exogenous agents, characterized in the acute stage by erythema, edema associated with a serous exudate between the cells of the epidermis (spongiosis) and an inflammatory infiltrate in the dermis, oozing and vesiculation, and crusting and scaling; and in the more chronic stages by lichenification or thickening or both, signs of excoriations, and hyperpigmentation or hypopigmentation or both. Atopic dermatitis is the most common type of dermatitis. Called also eczematous dermatitis. [EU]

Elastic: Susceptible of resisting and recovering from stretching, compression or distortion applied by a force. [EU]

Enzyme: A protein molecule that catalyses chemical reactions of other substances without itself being destroyed or altered upon completion of the reactions. Enzymes are classified according to the recommendations of the Nomenclature Committee of the International Union of Biochemistry. Each enzyme is assigned a recommended name and an Enzyme Commission (EC) number. They are divided into six main groups; oxidoreductases, transferases, hydrolases, lyases, isomerases, and ligases. [EU]

Epidermal: Pertaining to or resembling epidermis. Called also epidermic or epidermoid. [EU]

Epithelium: The covering of internal and external surfaces of the body, including the lining of vessels and other small cavities. It consists of cells joined by small amounts of cementing substances. Epithelium is classified into types on the basis of the number of layers deep and the shape of the superficial cells. [EU]

Erysipelas: An acute superficial form of cellulitis involving the dermal lymphatics, usually caused by infection with group A streptococci, and chiefly characterized by a peripherally spreading hot, bright red, edematous, brawny, infiltrated, and sharply circumscribed plaque with a raised indurated border. Formerly called St. Anthony's fire. [EU]

Erythrasma: A chronic, superficial bacterial infection of the skin involving the body folds and toe webs, sometimes becoming generalized, caused by Corynebacterium minutissimum, and characterized by the presence of sharply demarcated, dry, brown, slightly scaly, and slowly spreading patches. [EU]

Esterification: The process of converting an acid into an alkyl or aryl derivative. Most frequently the process consists of the reaction of an acid with an alcohol in the presence of a trace of mineral acid as catalyst or the reaction of an acyl chloride with an alcohol. Esterification can also be accomplished by enzymatic processes. [NIH]

Extracellular: Outside a cell or cells. [EU]

Fatal: Causing death, deadly; mortal; lethal. [EU]

Fissure: Any cleft or groove, normal or otherwise; especially a deep fold in the cerebral cortex which involves the entire thickness of the brain wall. [EU]

Fistula: An abnormal passage or communication, usually between two internal organs, or leading from an internal organ to the surface of the body; frequently designated according to the organs or parts with which it communicates, as anovaginal, brochocutaneous, hepatopleural, pulmonoperitoneal, rectovaginal, urethrovaginal, and the like. Such passages are frequently created experimentally for the purpose of obtaining body secretions for physiologic study. [EU]

Fluconazole: Triazole antifungal agent that is used to treat oropharyngeal candidiasis and cryptococcal meningitis in AIDS. [NIH]

Folliculitis: Inflammation of a follicle or follicles; used ordinarily in reference to hair follicles, but sometimes in relation to follicles of other kinds. [EU]

Genotype: The genetic constitution of the individual; the characterization of the genes. [NIH]

Granuloma: A relatively small nodular inflammatory lesion containing grouped mononuclear phagocytes, caused by infectious and noninfectious agents. [NIH]

Griseofulvin: An antifungal antibiotic. Griseofulvin may be given by mouth in the treatment of tinea infections. [NIH]

Groin: The external junctural region between the lower part of the abdomen and the thigh. [NIH]

Heredity: 1. the genetic transmission of a particular quality or trait from parent to offspring. 2. the genetic constitution of an individual. [EU]

Herpes: Any inflammatory skin disease caused by a herpesvirus and characterized by the formation of clusters of small vesicles. When used alone, the term may refer to herpes simplex or to herpes zoster. [EU]

Homeostasis: A tendency to stability in the normal body states (internal environment) of the organism. It is achieved by a system of control mechanisms activated by negative feedback; e.g. a high level of carbon dioxide in extracellular fluid triggers increased pulmonary ventilation, which in turn causes a decrease in carbon dioxide concentration. [EU]

Hormones: Chemical substances having a specific regulatory effect on the activity of a certain organ or organs. The term was originally applied to substances secreted by various endocrine glands and transported in the bloodstream to the target organs. It is sometimes extended to include those substances that are not produced by the endocrine glands but that have similar effects. [NIH]

Humoral: Of, relating to, proceeding from, or involving a bodily humour - now often used of endocrine factors as opposed to neural or somatic. [EU]

Hybridization: The genetic process of crossbreeding to produce a hybrid. Hybrid nucleic acids can be formed by nucleic acid hybridization of DNA and RNA molecules. Protein hybridization allows for hybrid proteins to be formed from polypeptide chains. [NIH]

Hydrogen: Hydrogen. The first chemical element in the periodic table. It has the atomic symbol H, atomic number 1, and atomic weight 1. It exists, under normal conditions, as a colorless, odorless, tasteless, diatomic gas. Hydrogen ions are protons. Besides the common H1 isotope, hydrogen exists as the stable isotope deuterium and the unstable, radioactive isotope tritium. [NIH]

Hyperkeratosis: 1. hypertrophy of the corneous layer of the skin. 2a. any of various conditions marked by hyperkeratosis. 2b. a disease of cattle marked by thickening and wringling of the hide and formation of papillary outgrowths on the buccal mucous membranes, often accompanied by watery discharge from eyes and nose, diarrhoea, loss of condition, and abortion of pregnant animals, and now believed to result from ingestion of the chlorinated naphthalene of various lubricating oils. [EU]

Hyperpigmentation: Excessive pigmentation of the skin, usually as a result of increased melanization of the epidermis rather than as a result of an increased number of melanocytes. Etiology is varied and the condition may arise from exposure to light, chemicals or other substances, or from a primary metabolic imbalance. [NIH]

Hyperthyroidism: 1. excessive functional activity of the thyroid gland. 2. the abnormal condition resulting from hyperthyroidism marked by increased metabolic rate, enlargement of the thyroid gland, rapid heart rate, high blood pressure, and various secondary symptoms. [EU]

Hypogonadism: A condition resulting from or characterized by abnormally decreased functional activity of the gonads, with retardation of growth and sexual development. [EU]

Hypopigmentation: A condition caused by a deficiency in melanin formation or a loss of pre-existing melanin or melanocytes. It can be complete or partial and may result from trauma, inflammation, and certain infections. [NIH]

Hypothyroidism: Deficiency of thyroid activity. In adults, it is most common in women and is characterized by decrease in basal metabolic rate, tiredness and lethargy, sensitivity to cold, and menstrual disturbances. If untreated, it progresses to full-blown myxoedema. In infants, severe hypothyroidism leads to cretinism. In juveniles, the manifestations are intermediate, with less severe mental and developmental retardation and only mild symptoms of the adult form. When due to pituitary deficiency of thyrotropin secretion it is called secondary hypothyroidism. [EU]

Ichthyosis: A group of cutaneous disorders characterized by increased or aberrant keratinization, resulting in noninflammatory scaling of the skin. Many different metaphors have been used to describe the appearance and texture of the skin in the various types and stages of ichthyosis, e.g. alligator, collodion, crocodile, fish, and porcupine skin. Most ichthyoses are genetically determined, while some may be acquired and develop in association with various systemic diseases or be a prominent feature in certain genetic syndromes. The term is commonly used alone to refer to i. vulgaris. [EU]

Immunohistochemistry: Histochemical localization of immunoreactive substances using labeled antibodies as reagents. [NIH]

Impetigo: A common superficial bacterial infection caused by staphylococcus aureus or group A beta-hemolytic streptococci. Characteristics include pustular lesions that rupture and discharge a thin, amber-colored fluid that dries and forms a crust. This condition is commonly located on the face, especially about the mouth and nose. [NIH]

Incubation: The development of an infectious disease from the entrance of the pathogen to the appearance of clinical symptoms. [EU]

Induction: The act or process of inducing or causing to occur, especially the production of a specific morphogenetic effect in the developing embryo through the influence of evocators or organizers, or the production of anaesthesia or unconsciousness by use of appropriate agents. [EU]

Infantile: Pertaining to an infant or to infancy. [EU]

Inflammation: A pathological process characterized by injury or destruction of tissues caused by a variety of cytologic and chemical reactions. It is usually manifested by typical signs of pain, heat, redness, swelling, and loss of function. [NIH]

Infusion: The therapeutic introduction of a fluid other than blood, as saline solution, solution, into a vein. [EU]

Innervation: 1. the distribution or supply of nerves to a part. 2. the supply of nervous energy or of nerve stimulus sent to a part. [EU]

Insulin: A protein hormone secreted by beta cells of the pancreas. Insulin plays a major role in the regulation of glucose metabolism, generally promoting the cellular utilization of glucose. It is also an important regulator of protein and lipid metabolism. Insulin is used as a drug to control insulin-dependent diabetes mellitus. [NIH]

Intertrigo: A superficial dermatitis occurring on apposed skin surfaces, such as the axillae, creases of the neck, intergluteal fold, groin, between the toes, and beneath pendulous breasts, with obesity being a predisposing factor, caused by moisture, friction, warmth, and sweat retention, and characterized by erythema, maceration, burning, itching, and sometimes erosions, fissures, and exudations and secondary infections. Called also eczema intertrigo. [EU]

Intramuscular: Within the substance of a muscle. [EU]

Iodine: A nonmetallic element of the halogen group that is represented by the atomic symbol I, atomic number 53, and atomic weight of 126.90. It is a nutritionally essential element, especially important in thyroid hormone synthesis. In solution, it has anti-infective properties and is used topically. [NIH]

Itraconazole: An antifungal agent that has been used in the treatment of histoplasmosis, blastomycosis, cryptococcal meningitis, and aspergillosis. [NIH]

Keloid: A sharply elevated, irregularly- shaped, progressively enlarging scar due to the formation of excessive amounts of collagen in the corium during connective tissue repair. [EU]

Keratitis: Inflammation of the cornea. [EU]

Kerosene: A refined petroleum fraction used as a fuel as well as a solvent. [NIH]

Ketoconazole: Broad spectrum antifungal agent used for long periods at high doses, especially in immunosuppressed patients. [NIH]

Leprosy: A chronic granulomatous infection caused by mycobacterium leprae. The granulomatous lesions are manifested in the skin, the mucous membranes, and the peripheral nerves. Two polar or principal types are lepromatous and tuberculoid. [NIH]

Lesion: Any pathological or traumatic discontinuity of tissue or loss of function of a part. [EU]

Lupus: A form of cutaneous tuberculosis. It is seen predominantly in women and typically involves the nasal, buccal, and conjunctival mucosa. [NIH]

Maceration: The softening of a solid by soaking. In histology, the softening of a tissue by soaking, especially in acids, until the connective tissue fibres are so dissolved that the tissue components can be teased apart. In obstetrics, the degenerative changes with discoloration and softening of tissues, and eventual disintegration, of a fetus retained in the uterus after its death. [EU]

Malignant: Tending to become progressively worse and to result in death. Having the properties of anaplasia, invasion, and metastasis; said of tumours. [EU]

Mechanoreceptors: Cells specialized to transduce mechanical stimuli and relay that information centrally in the nervous system. Mechanoreceptors include hair cells, which mediate hearing and balance, and the various somatosensory receptors, often with non-neural accessory structures. [NIH]

Mediator: An object or substance by which something is mediated, such as (1) a structure of the nervous system that transmits impulses eliciting a specific response; (2) a chemical substance (transmitter substance) that induces activity in an excitable tissue, such as nerve or muscle; or (3) a substance released from cells as the result of the interaction of antigen with antibody or by the action of antigen with a sensitized lymphocyte. [EU]

Melanocytes: Epidermal dendritic pigment cells which control long-term morphological color changes by alteration in their number or in the amount of pigment they produce and store in the pigment containing organelles called melanosomes. Melanophores are larger cells which do not exist in mammals. [NIH]

Melanoma: A tumour arising from the melanocytic system of the skin and other organs. When used alone the term refers to malignant melanoma. [EU]

Melanosomes: Melanin-containing organelles found in melanocytes and melanophores. [NIH]

Membrane: A thin layer of tissue which covers a surface, lines a cavity or divides a space or organ. [EU]

Methoxsalen: A naturally occurring furocoumarin compound found in several species of plants, including Psoralea corylifolia. It is a photoactive substance that forms DNA adducts in the presence of ultraviolet A irradiation. [NIH]

Miconazole: An imidazole antifungal agent that is used topically and by intravenous infusion. [NIH]

Microscopy: The application of microscope magnification to the study of materials that cannot be properly seen by the unaided eye. [NIH]

Modulator: A specific inductor that brings out characteristics peculiar to a definite region. [EU]

Molecular: Of, pertaining to, or composed of molecules : a very small mass of matter. [EU]

Myopia: That error of refraction in which rays of light entering the eye parallel to the optic axis are brought to a focus in front of the retina, as a result of the eyeball being too long from front to back (axial m.) or of an increased strength in refractive power of the media of the eye (index m.). Called also nearsightedness, because the near point is less distant than it is in emmetropia with an equal amplitude of accommodation. [EU]

Naltrexone: Derivative of noroxymorphone that is the N-cyclopropylmethyl congener of naloxone. It is a narcotic antagonist that is effective orally, longer lasting and more potent than naloxone, and has been proposed for the treatment of heroin addiction. The FDA has approved naltrexone for the treatment of alcohol dependence. [NIH]

Naphazoline: An adrenergic vasoconstrictor agent used as a decongestant. [NIH]

Natamycin: Amphoteric macrolide antifungal antibiotic from Streptomyces natalensis or S. chattanoogensis. It is used for a variety of fungal infections, mainly topically. [NIH]

Nausea: An unpleasant sensation, vaguely referred to the epigastrium and abdomen, and often culminating in vomiting. [EU]

Necrolysis: Separation or exfoliation of tissue due to necrosis. [EU]

Nephritis: Inflammation of the kidney; a focal or diffuse proliferative or destructive process which may involve the glomerulus, tubule, or interstitial renal tissue. [EU]

Neural: 1. pertaining to a nerve or to the nerves. 2. situated in the region of the spinal axis, as the neutral arch. [EU]

Neurology: A medical specialty concerned with the study of the structures, functions, and diseases of the nervous system. [NIH]

Neurons: The basic cellular units of nervous tissue. Each neuron consists of a body, an axon, and dendrites. Their purpose is to receive, conduct, and transmit impulses in the nervous system. [NIH]

Niacin: Water-soluble vitamin of the B complex occurring in various animal and plant tissues. Required by the body for the formation of coenzymes NAD and NADP. Has pellagra-curative, vasodilating, and antilipemic properties. [NIH]

Nystagmus: An involuntary, rapid, rhythmic movement of the eyeball, which may be horizontal, vertical, rotatory, or mixed, i.e., of two varieties. [EU]

Nystatin: Macrolide antifungal antibiotic complex produced by Streptomyces noursei, S. aureus, and other Streptomyces species. The biologically active components of the complex are nystatin A1, A2, and A3. [NIH]

Ocular: 1. of, pertaining to, or affecting the eye. 2. eyepiece. [EU]

Oligopeptides: Peptides composed of between two and twelve amino acids. [NIH]

Osteoporosis: Reduction in the amount of bone mass, leading to fractures after minimal trauma. [EU]

Papillomavirus: A genus of papovaviridae causing proliferation of the epithelium, which may lead to malignancy. A wide range of animals are infected including humans, chimpanzees, cattle, rabbits, dogs, and horses. [NIH]

Paraparesis: Mild to moderate loss of bilateral lower extremity motor function, which may be a manifestation of spinal cord diseases; peripheral nervous system diseases; muscular diseases; intracranial hypertension; parasagittal brain lesions; and other conditions. [NIH]

Percutaneous: Performed through the skin, as injection of radiopacque material in radiological examination, or the removal of tissue for biopsy accomplished by a needle. [EU]

Perinatal: Pertaining to or occurring in the period shortly before and after birth; variously defined as beginning with completion of the twentieth to twenty-eighth week of gestation and ending 7 to 28 days after birth. [EU]

Peroxidase: A hemeprotein from leukocytes. Deficiency of this enzyme leads to a hereditary disorder coupled with disseminated moniliasis. It catalyzes the conversion of a donor and peroxide to an oxidized donor and water. EC 1.11.1.7. [NIH]

Phenotype: The outward appearance of the individual. It is the product of interactions between genes and between the genotype and the environment. This includes the killer phenotype, characteristic of YEASTS. [NIH]

Photochemotherapy: Therapy using oral or topical photosensitizing agents with subsequent exposure to light. [NIH]

Photosensitivity: An abnormal cutaneous response involving the interaction between photosensitizing substances and sunlight or filtered or artificial light at wavelengths of 280-400 mm. There are two main types : photoallergy and photoxicity. [EU]

Phototherapy: Treatment of disease by exposure to light, especially by variously concentrated light rays or specific wavelengths. [NIH]

Pigmentation: 1. the deposition of colouring matter; the coloration or discoloration of a part by pigment. 2. coloration, especially abnormally increased coloration, by melanin. [EU]

Pityriasis: A name originally applied to a group of skin diseases characterized by the formation of fine, branny scales, but now used only with a modifier. [EU]

Placenta: A highly vascular fetal organ through which the fetus absorbs oxygen and other nutrients and excretes carbon dioxide and other wastes. It begins to form about the eighth day of gestation when the blastocyst adheres to the decidua. [NIH]

Polymorphic: Occurring in several or many forms; appearing in different forms at different stages of development. [EU]

Postnatal: Occurring after birth, with reference to the newborn. [EU]

Potassium: An element that is in the alkali group of metals. It has an atomic symbol K, atomic number 19, and atomic weight 39.10. It is the chief cation in the intracellular fluid of muscle and other cells. Potassium ion is a strong electrolyte and it plays a significant role in the regulation of fluid volume and maintenance of the water-electrolyte balance. [NIH]

Preclinical: Before a disease becomes clinically recognizable. [EU]

Precursor: Something that precedes. In biological processes, a substance from which another, usually more active or mature substance is formed. In clinical medicine, a sign or symptom that heralds another. [EU]

Propoxyphene: A narcotic analgesic structurally related to methadone. Only the dextro-isomer has an analgesic effect; the levo-isomer appears to exert an antitussive effect. [NIH]

Proteins: Polymers of amino acids linked by peptide bonds. The specific sequence of amino acids determines the shape and function of the protein. [NIH]

Proximal: Nearest; closer to any point of reference; opposed to distal. [EU]

Pruritus: 1. itching; an unpleasant cutaneous sensation that provokes the desire to rub or scratch the skin to obtain relief. 2. any of various conditions marked by itching, the specific site or type being indicated by a modifying term. [EU]

Psoriasis: A common genetically determined, chronic, inflammatory skin disease characterized by rounded erythematous, dry, scaling patches. The lesions have a predilection for nails, scalp, genitalia, extensor surfaces, and the lumbosacral region. Accelerated epidermopoiesis is considered to be the fundamental pathologic feature in psoriasis. [NIH]

Pustular: Pertaining to or of the nature of a pustule; consisting of pustules (= a visible collection of pus within or beneath the epidermis). [EU]

Receptor: 1. a molecular structure within a cell or on the surface characterized by (1) selective binding of a specific substance and (2) a specific physiologic effect that accompanies the binding, e.g., cell-surface receptors for peptide hormones, neurotransmitters, antigens, complement fragments, and immunoglobulins and cytoplasmic receptors for steroid hormones. 2. a sensory nerve terminal that responds to stimuli of various kinds. [EU]

Recombinant: 1. a cell or an individual with a new combination of genes not found together in either parent; usually applied to linked genes. [EU]

Rectal: Pertaining to the rectum (= distal portion of the large intestine). [EU]

Regeneration: The natural renewal of a structure, as of a lost tissue or part. [EU]

Retina: The ten-layered nervous tissue membrane of the eye. It is continuous with the optic nerve and receives images of external objects and transmits visual impulses to the brain. Its outer surface is in contact with the choroid and the inner surface with the vitreous body. The outer-most layer is pigmented, whereas the inner nine layers are transparent. [NIH]

Retinoids: Derivatives of vitamin A. Used clinically in the treatment of severe cystic acne, psoriasis, and other disorders of keratinization. Their possible use in the prophylaxis and treatment of cancer is being actively explored. [NIH]

Retinopathy: 1. retinitis (= inflammation of the retina). 2. retinosis (= degenerative, noninflammatory condition of the retina). [EU]

Rhodopsin: A photoreceptor protein found in retinal rods. It is a complex formed by the binding of retinal, the oxidized form of retinol, to the protein opsin and undergoes a series of complex reactions in response to visible light resulting in the transmission of nerve impulses to the brain. [NIH]

Riboflavin: Nutritional factor found in milk, eggs, malted barley, liver, kidney, heart, and leafy vegetables. The richest natural source is yeast. It occurs in the free form only in the retina of the eye, in whey, and in urine; its principal forms in tissues and cells are as FMN and FAD. [NIH]

Sarcoma: A tumour made up of a substance like the embryonic connective tissue; tissue composed of closely packed cells embedded in a fibrillar or homogeneous substance. Sarcomas are often highly malignant. [EU]

Sclerosis: A induration, or hardening; especially hardening of a part from inflammation and in diseases of the interstitial substance. The term is used chiefly for such a hardening of the nervous system due to hyperplasia of the connective tissue or to designate hardening of the blood vessels. [EU]

Selenium: An element with the atomic symbol Se, atomic number 34, and atomic weight 78.96. It is an essential micronutrient for mammals and other animals but is toxic in large amounts. Selenium protects intracellular structures against oxidative damage. It is an essential component of glutathione peroxidase. [NIH]

Serum: The clear portion of any body fluid; the clear fluid moistening serous membranes. 2. blood serum; the clear liquid that separates from blood on clotting. 3. immune serum; blood serum from an immunized animal used for passive immunization; an antiserum; antitoxin, or antivenin. [EU]

Spastic: 1. of the nature of or characterized by spasms. 2. hypertonic, so that the muscles are stiff and the movements awkward. 3. a person exhibiting spasticity, such as occurs in spastic paralysis or in cerebral palsy. [EU]

Species: A taxonomic category subordinate to a genus (or subgenus) and superior to a subspecies or variety, composed of individuals possessing common characters distinguishing them from other categories of individuals of the same taxonomic level. In taxonomic nomenclature, species are designated by the genus name followed by a Latin or Latinized adjective or noun. [EU]

Spectrum: A charted band of wavelengths of electromagnetic vibrations obtained by refraction and diffraction. By extension, a measurable range of activity, such as the range of bacteria affected by an antibiotic (antibacterial s.) or the complete range of manifestations of a disease. [EU]

Squamous: Scaly, or platelike. [EU]

Suction: The removal of secretions, gas or fluid from hollow or tubular organs or cavities by means of a tube and a device that acts on negative pressure. [NIH]

Sulfur: An element that is a member of the chalcogen family. It has an atomic symbol S, atomic number 16, and atomic weight 32.066. It is found in the amino acids cysteine and methionine. [NIH]

Sunburn: An injury to the skin causing erythema, tenderness, and sometimes blistering and resulting from excessive exposure to the sun. The reaction is produced by the ultraviolet radiation in sunlight. [NIH]

Surgical: Of, pertaining to, or correctable by surgery. [EU]

Thyroxine: An amino acid of the thyroid gland which exerts a stimulating effect on thyroid metabolism. [NIH]

Topical: Pertaining to a particular surface area, as a topical anti-infective applied to a certain area of the skin and affecting only the area to which it is applied. [EU]

Toxin: A poison; frequently used to refer specifically to a protein produced by some higher plants, certain animals, and pathogenic bacteria, which is highly toxic for other living organisms. Such substances are differentiated from the simple chemical poisons and the vegetable alkaloids by their high molecular weight and antigenicity. [EU]

Tretinoin: An important regulator of gene expression, particularly during growth and development and in neoplasms. Retinoic acid derived from maternal vitamin A is essential for normal gene expression during embryonic development and either a deficiency or an excess can be teratogenic. It is also a topical dermatologic agent which is used in the treatment of psoriasis, acne vulgaris, and several other skin diseases. It has also been approved for use in promyelocytic leukemia. [NIH]

Uveitis: An inflammation of part or all of the uvea, the middle (vascular) tunic of the eye, and commonly involving the other tunics (the sclera and cornea, and the retina). [EU]

Vaccination: The introduction of vaccine into the body for the purpose of inducing immunity. Coined originally to apply to the injection of smallpox vaccine, the term has come to mean any immunizing procedure in which vaccine is injected. [EU]

Vaccine: A suspension of attenuated or killed microorganisms (bacteria, viruses, or rickettsiae), administered for the prevention, amelioration or treatment of infectious diseases. [EU]

Vaccinia: The cutaneous and sometimes systemic reactions associated with vaccination with smallpox vaccine. [EU]

Varicella: Chicken pox. [EU]

Vasculitis: Inflammation of a vessel, angiitis. [EU]

Vestibular: Pertaining to or toward a vestibule. In dental anatomy, used to refer to the tooth surface directed toward the vestibule of the mouth. [EU]

Viral: Pertaining to, caused by, or of the nature of virus. [EU]

Viruses: Minute infectious agents whose genomes are composed of DNA or RNA, but not both. They are characterized by a lack of independent metabolism and the inability to replicate outside living host cells. [NIH]

Vitiligo: A disorder consisting of areas of macular depigmentation, commonly on extensor aspects of extremities, on the face or neck, and in skin folds. Age of onset is often in young adulthood and the condition tends to progress gradually with lesions enlarging and extending until a quiescent state is reached. [NIH]

Warts: Benign epidermal proliferations or tumors; some are viral in origin. [NIH]

Xanthoma: A tumour composed of lipid-laden foam cells, which are histiocytes containing cytoplasmic lipid material. Called also xanthelasma. [EU]

General Dictionaries and Glossaries

While the above glossary is essentially complete, the dictionaries listed here cover virtually all aspects of medicine, from basic words and phrases to more advanced terms (sorted alphabetically by title; hyperlinks provide rankings, information and reviews at Amazon.com):

- **Dictionary of Medical Acronymns & Abbreviations** by Stanley Jablonski (Editor), Paperback, 4th edition (2001), Lippincott Williams & Wilkins Publishers, ISBN: 1560534605,
  http://www.amazon.com/exec/obidos/ASIN/1560534605/icongroupinterna

- **Dictionary of Medical Terms : For the Nonmedical Person (Dictionary of Medical Terms for the Nonmedical Person, Ed 4)** by Mikel A. Rothenberg, M.D, et al, Paperback - 544 pages, 4th edition (2000), Barrons Educational Series, ISBN: 0764112015,
  http://www.amazon.com/exec/obidos/ASIN/0764112015/icongroupinterna

- **A Dictionary of the History of Medicine** by A. Sebastian, CD-Rom edition (2001), CRC Press-Parthenon Publishers, ISBN: 185070368X,
  http://www.amazon.com/exec/obidos/ASIN/185070368X/icongroupinterna

- **Dorland's Illustrated Medical Dictionary (Standard Version)** by Dorland, et al, Hardcover - 2088 pages, 29th edition (2000), W B Saunders Co, ISBN: 0721662544,
  http://www.amazon.com/exec/obidos/ASIN/0721662544/icongroupinterna

- **Dorland's Electronic Medical Dictionary** by Dorland, et al, Software, 29th Book & CD-Rom edition (2000), Harcourt Health Sciences, ISBN: 0721694934,
  http://www.amazon.com/exec/obidos/ASIN/0721694934/icongroupinterna

- **Dorland's Pocket Medical Dictionary (Dorland's Pocket Medical Dictionary, 26th Ed)** Hardcover - 912 pages, 26th edition (2001), W B Saunders Co, ISBN: 0721682812,
  http://www.amazon.com/exec/obidos/ASIN/0721682812/icongroupintern a/103-4193558-7304618

- **Melloni's Illustrated Medical Dictionary (Melloni's Illustrated Medical Dictionary, 4th Ed)** by Melloni, Hardcover, 4th edition (2001), CRC Press-Parthenon Publishers, ISBN: 85070094X,
  http://www.amazon.com/exec/obidos/ASIN/85070094X/icongroupinterna

- **Stedman's Electronic Medical Dictionary Version 5.0 (CD-ROM for Windows and Macintosh, Individual)** by Stedmans, CD-ROM edition (2000), Lippincott Williams & Wilkins Publishers, ISBN: 0781726328, http://www.amazon.com/exec/obidos/ASIN/0781726328/icongroupinterna

- **Stedman's Medical Dictionary** by Thomas Lathrop Stedman, Hardcover - 2098 pages, 27th edition (2000), Lippincott, Williams & Wilkins, ISBN: 068340007X, http://www.amazon.com/exec/obidos/ASIN/068340007X/icongroupinterna

- **Tabers Cyclopedic Medical Dictionary (Thumb Index)** by Donald Venes (Editor), et al, Hardcover - 2439 pages, 19th edition (2001), F A Davis Co, ISBN: 0803606540, http://www.amazon.com/exec/obidos/ASIN/0803606540/icongroupinterna

INDEX

Printed in the United States
28809LVS00001B/35